Praise for
The Wild & Weedy Apothecary

When you read this book, you'll feel like you're out in the fields
on a beautiful spring day with a knowledgeable and entertaining
friend. If you have ever wanted to know more about the wonder of
wild herbs, Doreen will lead the way.

Dr. Deborah Duchon
Cultural anthropologist, former publisher of *The Wild
Foods Forum*, and guest on FoodNetwork's *Good Eats*
with Alton Brown

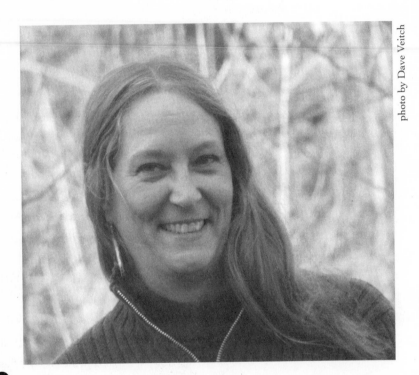

DOREEN SHABABY gardens, writes, sings, cooks, and crafts from her home in northern Idaho. Her articles, book reviews, recipes, and poetry have appeared in several publications. Doreen grew up in Chicago and moved to Idaho as a teen, where she began her study of wild edible plants and herbal healing, and eventually learned to cook. Later on, she self-published a quarterly called *Wild & Weedy—A Journal of Herbology*, and continues to network with others on behalf of herbs and herbalism, and other healing arts. A mother and grandmother, sister, auntie, and wife, Doreen makes her home with her husband, fine woodworker Dave Veitch, and their furry four-leggeds.

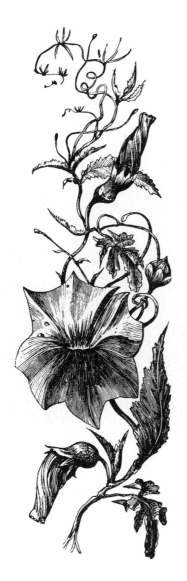

The
Wild & Weedy
APOTHECARY

An A to Z Book of
Herbal Concoctions,
Recipes & Remedies
Practical Know-How
—*and*—
Food for the Soul

Doreen Shababy

Llewellyn Publications / *Woodbury, Minnesota*

FIRST EDITION
First Printing, 2010

Book design by Rebecca Zins
Cover design by Adrienne Zimiga
Cover florals © 1997 Elizabeth Dowle/Quarto, Inc./Artville, LLC
Interior floral elements © 1990 by Dover Publications, Inc.,
from *Old-Fashioned Floral Designs CD-ROM and Book*

Llewellyn is a registered trademark of Llewellyn Worldwide, Ltd.

Library of Congress Cataloging-in-Publication Data
Shababy, Doreen, 1958-
    The wild & weedy apothecary : an A to Z book of herbal concoctions,
recipes & remedies practical know-how and food for the soul / Doreen
Shababy.—1st ed.
        p. cm.
    Includes bibliographical references and index.
    ISBN 978-0-7387-1907-8
    1. Cookery (Herbs) 2. Herbs—Therapeutic use. I. Title. II. Title:
Wild and weedy apothecary.
    TX819.H4S485 2010
    641.6'57—dc22
                                        2009051928

Llewellyn Worldwide does not participate in, endorse, or have any authority or
responsibility concerning private business transactions between our authors and
the public.
    All mail addressed to the author is forwarded, but the publisher cannot, unless
specifically instructed by the author, give out an address or phone number.
    Any Internet references contained in this work are current at publication time,
but the publisher cannot guarantee that a specific location will continue to be
maintained. Please refer to the publisher's website for links to authors' websites
and other sources.

Llewellyn Publications
A Division of Llewellyn Worldwide, Ltd.
2143 Wooddale Drive, Dept. 978-0-7387-1907-8
Woodbury, MN 55125-2989
www.llewellyn.com

Printed in the United States of America

Acknowledgments

To my family, friends, relatives, kith and kin, I thank you most sincerely. You all know who you are, and I am forever grateful for your continued encouragement and support. I have spoken with many of you about this project for quite some time, and I thank you for hanging in there with me to see its fruition.

The East Bonner County Library and staff deserves my years-long appreciation for accessing books for me from libraries from Alaska to Arizona, and for all the books they acquired seemingly at my request. They have always been and continue to be most gracious, and my research was greatly enhanced by this congenial relationship, for which I am so thankful. I ❤ my library!

Many thanks to the following individuals for their support in helping me create my original journal and for the inspiration to continue the work and complete this book: local instigator Diane Newcomer and trusted science counselor Edie Kinucan; writers and contributors Robin Klein, Julie Summers, Joy Bittner, Beverly Red, Zella Bardsley, Kahlee "RootWoman" Keene, Jackie Ramirez, and Harvest McCampbell; fellow herb-zine editors James Troy, Deb Duchon, and Vickie Schufer; Debbie Boots, wild food expert and instructor long before it was cool; Debi Richardson for production refinery; *Aha!* elf Sara Wallace; origami apprentice Rose Shababy, for unrelenting support; ink-master and expert idea-interpreter Mike Fellin; computer benefactor and proud mom Dorothy Dunn; and beloved wood wizard Dave Veitch. I also want to thank all my brothers and sisters, those in-laws and outlaws of my life on whom I know I can always depend. I thank my women's circle for cheering me on. (If I've missed someone, it is purely unintentional.)

A jovial twirl of the wooden spoon to the following people for sharing their recipes with me and allowing me to include them in this book: Carol Romagnano, Irene Daanen, Deanna McDevitt, Lynn "Bullhead" Reese, Valerie Usdrowski, Lisa "Lulu" DeGrace, Joel Aispuro, Jeannine Johnson, Sue Rider, Jayne Schaper, Joy Bittner, Debbie "Coyote Woman" Mann, and Jeannie Weatherford. I have done my best to give credit where credit is due.

My old friend Edie passed away while I was preparing the manuscript for this book, and I'm very sorry she couldn't have seen the completed work. She has been a counsel to me from the beginning.

A special thank you to Carrie Obry and Rebecca Zins, and all of Llewellyn Publications, for having confidence in my work and for encouraging me to be Me.

Each and every one of you has been a teacher to me in your own way; I am so blessed.

This book is dedicated to my grandchildren, Quinton & Leeland and Miranda & Justine, and all the young ones, so they have some place to begin their journey. May this book be a springboard for their curiosity and imagination.

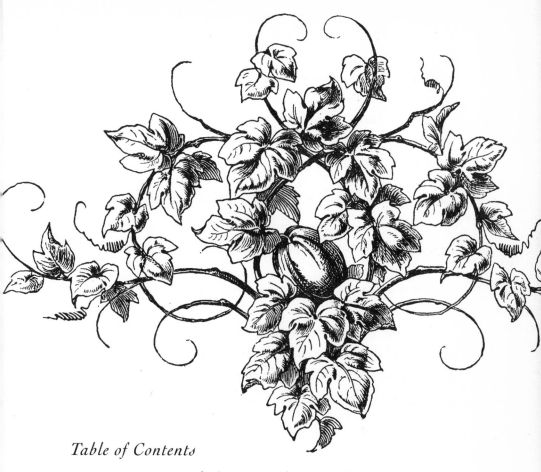

Table of Contents

. . . .

₽ART 1
How to Use This Book

₽ART 2
Encyclopedia of Recipes & Remedies

On Taking Herbal Remedies

I want to explain my use of the term *medicine*. I do not necessarily use the term the way a medical doctor would, such as in the case of prescription drugs or such, or even things like vitamins and supplements and so on. To me, medicine means something different, beyond the mere physical to a more heightened sense of awareness and being—awareness in the act of preparing a soothing pot of tea, or awareness in making a batch of herbal healing salve for friends and family, to see them through the bumps and bruises of life. This book isn't about medical medicine; it's about spirit medicine, the kind you get when you pick strawberries with your children and see happy faces at the potluck as your friends discover fresh dinner rolls with honey butter. The side effects of this type of medicine are completely positive.

I salute the discoveries of science, from microcosm to macrocosm, and am no stranger to a microscope or a telescope. I do wash my hands a lot in the kitchen, but not with antibacterial soap—for gosh sakes, plain old hand soap is as clean as need be.

If you have a medical condition that needs monitoring by a physician, you should ask him or her about the remedies in this book before trying them on yourself. I have confidence that they are safe when used as instructed. I have taken extra consideration in noting when a recipe, remedy, or ingredient is inappropriate for babies or pregnant women. You are responsible for your own personal choices, and I won't be held responsible if you wander from the parameters of my instructions.

Introduction

Welcome to the wild and weedy apothecary, a place where herbs hang in bunches from the rafters, potions brew in glass jars on the medicine hutch, and there's always time for a cup of fragrant tea. I invite you to pull up a chair, savor a steaming bowl of soup, and enjoy your visit.

I have pursued an empirical education in herbal healing for over thirty years, especially home remedies, with emphasis on local wild plants and those plants I can grow myself. In the late 1980s, I self-published a small—what I call "kitchen table"—magazine called *Wild & Weedy—A Journal of Herbology*. Originally typed on an old manual typewriter, my dear baby of a chapbook took root and blossomed.

It was a terrific learning experience for me. Feature articles included the study of wild plants for food and medicine, organic gardening, seasonal celebrations, prose and poetry, and always recipes and remedies, some of which were gleaned from other herb books or given to me by generous mothers and homemakers—the original herbalists—desiring to share this information. Many of us could see that these "old ways" were valid, and we wanted to pass them on to the next generation. I also thought it was important to write about what I had personally experienced with each plant.

I also traded subscriptions with other magazines, which was quite a bonus. Even though *W & W* had a small circulation, I received inquiries from people all over the world—from the director of an indigenous plant studies program in Brazil to native plant growers in Poland, from the Friends of the Trees Society in north central Washington to the

University of Idaho. *W & W* was even included in Some 'Zines, an exhibit of small and "underground" publications displayed at Boise State University in 1992. Many people were willing to share information, and I was constantly amazed at how my little journal got around.

In between the magazine and continuing personal studies, I taught classes for making herbal body products such as salves and lotions, and I sold these along with fresh herbs and herbal seasoning blends at farmer's markets and barter fairs. I started taking folks out on guided "weed walks" for plant identification, either on their property or on forest trails. This was a real challenge for me, as I am much more comfortable at the stove or computer keyboard than leading the pack! Although I have never taken a formal course in herbalism, I have participated in many a bull session in the herb garden as well as the forest with the women and men who helped round out my book learnin' with some useful, practical knowledge. Class is always in session.

Enter the kitchen. There is a certainty in my family that, even when the fridge is empty and the cupboard bare, I can not only make a meal, I can make it taste like I had all the ingredients in the world to choose from. It's comments like that which encourage my culinary self-confidence, and I constantly broaden my tastes and curiosity. Don't get me wrong—I'm not a fancy-pants chef creating three-story condos on a dessert plate, but I do consider myself an excellent cook, with a passion for good, wholesome, flavorful food. When I cook, I like to imagine that the soul is satisfied too. As aromas fill the air with anticipation, I consider it a blessing to be skilled at preparing delicious food. My family and friends appreciate it too. The following story is a case in point.

Many years ago, my brother came up from Florida to visit my mountain home in Idaho. Recalling my previous cooking ability, he asked, "Do you still burn water?"—at which point I proceeded to knock everyone's socks off with a complete fried chicken dinner—you know, the coronary feast including mashed taters'n'gravy, sweet corn, biscuits, wild green salad, and so on, followed by a wild (yes, wild) strawberry shortcake, with berries my daughter helped pick. Did I mention that I prepared this meal on a wood stove? We didn't have electricity "up there" at the time, and I believe this was a major turning point in my culinary prowess; I even impressed myself!

The Great Chicken Dinner is just one of the stories that have emerged from the wild and weedy apothecary. In this book, I have used my favorite recipes and remedies from the journal and rounded them out with an A to Z of healthy, helpful ideas that I trust you will find appealing as well as informative. My intention isn't merely to instruct—and I promise to be as clear as consommé concerning home remedies and wild plants. But because I enjoy gardening and the great outdoors, I also hope to share the delight I feel when I brush my hand through the lemon thyme or pick the ingredients for a snappy salsa fresh from the garden. I want you to know what it smells like in the spring forest, and I hope to inspire you to find out for yourself. Here, you'll find a celebration of the wild, get your toes wet on seasonal garden tours, and catch a glimpse into my culinary family album. You'll also observe the influence of friends and ideas past and present. I share the basic techniques I use in the wild and weedy apothecary, along with my version of a well-stocked pantry and "medicine cabinet." Some of the items are in both places; some of the ideas will surprise you.

I follow a basic preventative approach to health by eating good-quality food and using herbs for seasoning. My emphasis on what to eat is based on whole, wild, homegrown, handmade, and delicious foods. As a kid in the 1960s, I certainly consumed my share of Kool-Aid and tuna casserole (and I'm not opposed to a bacon cheeseburger now and then), but growing up I was also exposed to no small variety of homey, ethnic dishes such as my Polish gramma's apricot kolachkes, my Italian gramma's spaghetti gravy with stuffed calamari, and my dad's Lebanese tradition of roast turkey stuffed with rice, pine nuts, and cinnamon (where do you think a name like Shababy came from?). My mom knew where to find Chicago's best barbecue ribs, and she was no stranger to the hook-and-worm end of a fishing pole. Each summer, we grew a small vegetable garden in our little backyard, with tomatoes, bell peppers, beans, cucumbers, and sweet corn—ohhh, that Illinois sweet corn. We lived as an extended family, like people used to do, and from there I observed my Gramma Lil's green thumb tending her perennial flowers and rose garden out front in addition to the veggies out back. When we moved to Idaho, wild plants (and the music of John Denver!) became my best friends. It was easy to lose myself in the sights and sounds of the forest and meadows that surrounded me, observing the plants and animals around my new home. I wanted to know all about them, and now I want to share some of what I've learned with you.

This book emphasizes our collective experience with herbs and what they can do for you. While there are plenty of fun recipes to cook and share with family and friends, *The Wild & Weedy Apothecary* is primarily an herbal. Full instructions are included on how to make all the home remedies you might need for common use—calming syrups for coughs and colds, cooling compresses for bumps and bruises, soothing elixirs for rest and relaxation. The cooking instructions have been carefully worked out for clarity and ease. I have included an extensive bibliography for further reference.

However, there is no one right way to read and use *The Wild & Weedy Apothecary*. You can open the book to any chapter you wish and find something useful and interesting. And because this herbal is also about food, you could go to the list of recipes by category on page 335 and see what inspires you. I want you to have fun on your visit, and at the same time, I hope to impart information that is of practical use to you.

I'm still working to grow all my own herbs, with nasturtiums galore and enough basil to make freezer pesto. Each year's batch of homemade salsa tastes a little different from the last, with names like golden cha-cha sauce and tomato sunrise (yes, I name my food). I like a good sharp knife and stacks of wooden plates, bowls, and spoons. When I cook, I fling food like a Cuisinart gone berserk; my stove is a disaster area. I sneak in dried nettles wherever I can get away with it, including my dogs' food. I also make and take my own remedies.

Once you step into *The Wild & Weedy Apothecary*, I believe you'll want to visit again. May you find comfort in the familiar and excitement in the new.

Love, peace, and blessings,

Doreen Shababy
SPRING 2009

"I suppose you could make medicines that would be distasteful, but it seems ever so much better to let your kitchen become your apothecary."

—Jeanne Rose, author and herbalist,
Jeanne Rose's Herbal Guide to Inner Health

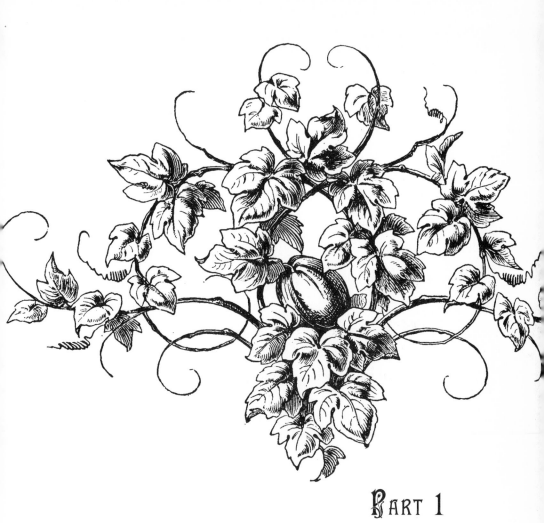

Part 1

How to
Use This Book

The Kitchen Apothecary

The purpose of this first chapter is to familiarize you with the various methods of preparing herbs for home remedies; it's a definitive how-to section. This is one of the most important chapters in the book, because it is referred to so often in other chapters. The instructions are clear and simple. Some methods use fresh herbs and some use dried. None of the ingredients or equipment is strange or expensive, and most things you already have on hand. You will find recommended dosages for each remedy in the text, and when used according to the instructions, a little common sense, and perhaps an elementary knowledge of North American herbs (should you choose to forage your own), these recipes are safe. I have also included a list of equipment and supplies that are the basic components used in many of the remedies, not counting the herbs. I have tried to make this book as user-friendly as possible.

Which brings me to another important point regarding this book. *The Wild & Weedy Apothecary* is not an herbal identification book, it's about what to do with the herbs once you have them. Check out the extensive bibliography at the back of the book for a list of field guides and other relevant handbooks. You will need to use guides appropriate to your region, and the best place to find these kinds of books is your local library.

This is also a book about using herbs for eating well and having fun with your food (I highly recommend singing and laughing at the dinner table). Packed with vitamins and minerals, herbs are a healthy and flavorful way to boost the food value of a simple bowl of rice or noodles without much fuss. There's more nutrition in a pinch of parsley or cilantro than a whole bowl of lettuce, but how much better they look and taste when combined as a salad.

Please note that some herbs are inappropriate for babies, children, and pregnant or nursing women. Throughout this book, I have explicitly noted the ingredients that fall into that category. When in doubt, please ask your midwife, a knowledgeable herbalist, or a competent health-care practitioner.

Equipment and Tools

As mentioned above, none of the equipment used in the kitchen apothecary need be strange or expensive. When I think about it, nearly all my tools and utensils are multi-taskers. The list is simple, common, and familiar, and substitutions are easy to locate. Do not hesitate to recycle used jars and such—just be sure to clean them thoroughly. What follows is a list of tools I consistently use for cooking and herb-crafting; I doubt you'll have to run out and buy anything special to create the recipes or remedies in this book.

- baskets, wide and shallow, for drying herbs
- blender or food processor (I have a mini processor, which is a great little tool)
- box grater
- canning jars, preferably wide-mouth quarts, pints and half-pints, with lids
- cast-iron skillets (I realize this is not so common)
- cheesecloth or other appropriate fabric, for filtering liquids
- chef's knife and paring knife, and a way to keep them sharp
- citrus juicer or reamer
- coffee or spice grinder (not necessary but nice)
- colander or sieve for larger foods
- cups and mugs for tea, and bowls for soup
- cutting boards

- dropper bottles (get these at your pharmacy or herb supplier)
- food dehydrator (useful but not necessary)
- freezer bags and other storage containers
- funnels
- glass baking dishes
- large kettle for making broth and sterilizing bottles
- kitchen twine, rubber bands
- measuring cups and spoons
- mixing bowls, different sizes
- mortar and pestle
- rubber spatula, and also the kind you flip with
- saucepans with lids—stainless steel, enamelware, or heat-resistant glass
- slow-cooker (the mini version isn't necessary but it's oh-so-useful)
- spray bottles (can be recycled)
- storage jars, bottles and canisters, airtight (these can be recycled)
- stove and oven
- strainers in various sizes, for tea and other liquids
- tea kettle (although a saucepan will certainly do for boiling water)
- teapot for serving
- teaspoons, the kind you stir with
- towels and clean rags, for cleaning
- vegetable peeler
- waxed paper and plastic wrap
- weight scale (an inexpensive postal scale is fine)
- wooden spoons and chopsticks

If you are just starting out on your own and stocking your first kitchen, this list may seem daunting, but you can find a good number of these items at thrift stores and yard sales, which is where I found some of my own kitchenware. When the kitchen is your shop, you find a way. I do recommend quality over quantity, especially concerning knives.

Herbal Remedy Ingredients

These are items I keep in stock for making herbal home remedies. They are common and easy to come by at familiar places such as your local grocery store or pharmacy, farmer's market, or natural food store.

- almond oil
- beeswax
- castile soap, preferably liquid
- cocoa butter
- honey
- olive oil
- pure grain alcohol (can substitute with 100-proof vodka)
- sea salt
- vinegar, especially apple cider vinegar
- vitamin E oil
- water, preferably filtered or spring
- prepared witch hazel

As you can see, nothing on this list is exotic. It really needn't be— that's the beauty of the kitchen apothecary. You see, you're not setting up a laboratory, this is your home, a place for nurturing and rejuvenation. You don't need a bunch of multi-syllabic chemical ingredients floating around in your personal body care products. While children shouldn't get hold of a few obvious ingredients, they remain family-friendly when properly prepared and administered by a responsible adult.

Read all instructions thoroughly before embarking on a project so you are ready for possible contingencies, and have all your equipment and ingredients located and at the ready. But don't worry, the recipes and remedies in this book are very doable; in fact, most are downright fun, and children can help with many of them.

Dried Simples

This means, simply, dried herbs used for teas (also known as *tisanes*, a lovely French term), infusions, or decoctions. The difference between these terms lies in the quantity of dried plant material in relation to the amount of water, and how long it is steeped or simmered. It does not refer to black tea such as Darjeeling or oolong, which is a whole cult unto itself. Never use aluminum or iron to prepare any herbal remedy, as these metals will cause an unfavorable reaction with the herbs. Instead, use stainless steel, enamelware, or heat-tempered glass to prepare your brews, and use good water. If you have chlorinated municipal water, you may wish to invest in a water filter for your regular drinking water.

HERB TEA — For a simple herbal beverage, or tisane, use one rounded teaspoon (not necessarily a measuring teaspoon but the kind you stir with) dried, crushed plant material or two teaspoons fresh to a teacup or mug full of boiling water, steeping (soaking) for only a few minutes. You may wish to steep in a jar (or teapot — hey, there's an idea!) to make it easier to strain, then pour into the cup and sweeten if desired. Two to three cups a day is not too much tea, although most are diuretic to some degree. There are a multitude of herbs to use as tea such as spearmint, chamomile, or nettles, and it's fun to experiment with flavorful combinations. Check out page 264, "T is for Tea," and try out a few of my own favorites.

HERBAL INFUSION — An herbal infusion is a strong tea used as a remedy. Use one ounce dried plant material (usually leaves or flowers) and add to one pint boiling water, cover, remove from heat, and steep ten to fifteen minutes. The herb itself is not boiled. Strain and serve. This will be your dose of medicinal tea, and you might take only a few sips at a time, depending on the remedy. Some instructions note whether to drink hot or cold and the time of day for best effect.

HERBAL DECOCTION — For a decoction, a strong medicinal tea that is simmered, use one ounce dried plant material (usually a tougher part of the plant, such as the root, bark, twig, seed, or berry) to one pint water, then cover and simmer for about fifteen minutes, depending on the plant parts and desired strength.

In practical use, an ounce of dried plant material can be quite a large volume — up to a cup. I find that if I need a lung congestion remedy, for instance, a good, strong, hot cup or two of, say, mullein leaf tea combined with some mint is just as remedial as the herbal infusion. Generally speaking, teas and infusions extract the volatile oils and water-soluble components from the plant, while decoctions extract the "bitters" and other components. Most herbs can be used fresh for teas, but some must actually be dried and aged to make them useful or safe, such as the laxative herb cascara. Remember the rules about herbs and pregnancy: when in doubt, don't.

Herbal Poultice, or Plaster

This method of using herbs employs moisture and/or heat for the healing action. They are used to heal bruises, reduce inflammation, break up congestion, and as a drawing agent for slivers or infections.

SIMPLE POULTICE — One way to make a poultice — the easiest way, in fact — is to use fresh herbs such as chickweed, self-heal (heal-all), violet leaf, or other gentle emollient herbs, and either mash them up in a bowl using a fork or a wooden spoon, buzz them in the blender, or chew them into a pulp (this is especially useful out on the trail), and apply directly to the affected area. A piece of cabbage, plantain, or other large, non-irritating leaf, carefully secured with a strip of gauze ribbon, holds the poultice in place. Alternatively, you can just sit still for a few minutes while the poultice is doing its thing and not worry about covering it, and then be on your merry way; this is what I've done for bee stings on the hiking trail (if you are allergic to bee stings, you already know what you have to do). Chickweed (*Stellaria media*), a common garden "weed," makes a very good poultice for infected splinters.

COMPOUND PLASTER — Another type of poultice, or plaster, is made by grinding the selected dried herb, mixing it into an equal amount of bran, oatmeal, or flaxseed meal (or some sort of neutral medium), then adding enough very hot water to make a wet paste. The amounts needed depend on the area you are covering. Spread this on a warm, moistened piece of muslin or cheesecloth, sized to lay over the affected area, then cover with another piece of dry cloth. A ginger compress is a traditional Chinese remedy for pulmonary complaints (chest), kidney blockage (middle back), and menstrual cramps (abdomen and lower back). The herbal plaster is less commonly used than the simple poultice or herb compress, partly because it's more complicated and partly because it's difficult to apply on one's self. Some plasters can be made without the bran and just the plant material, such as an apple plaster for sunburn.

HERB COMPRESS — A compress is similar to a plaster but much simpler and easier to use. A strong, hot infusion of the selected herb is prepared. Soft cloths or towels are dipped into the tea, then wrung out and applied to the affected area. Keep the "patient" warm by covering with them with a towel or blanket. Some compresses should be cool, such as for sunburn or sprains. Of course, some conditions such as a broken bone would require cold applications, at least until emergency medical treatment becomes available; there must be reason and common sense used when treating ourselves, and knowing our limitations is part of that.

Herbal Tinctures

An alcohol-based tincture using fresh or dried herbs is a method of concentrating the medicinal qualities of herbs for internal use. One terrific benefit of herb tinctures is that they keep just about forever.

HERBAL TINCTURE — These are prepared by steeping approximately one ounce dried or four ounces fresh plant material, chopped or gently crushed (do not powder) in one pint (or enough liquid to cover the herb) good-quality vodka in a fresh, clean jar. Label and date. The tincture should steep about two weeks — longer for tougher material. While some herbals might suggest brandy or gin, I prefer 100-proof vodka (which is exactly 50 percent alcohol and 50 percent water) for most fresh flowers, leaves, and dried herbs. I choose pure grain alcohol or Everclear for fresh roots or other tough or resinous plant material, such as cottonwood buds; if you can't find Everclear, try 151-proof rum.

Since tinctures are concentrated, the dose is taken in drops (not droppers-full), usually from ten to thirty drops per adult dose, according to the herbs and the body weight of the person. Add the drops to water so they don't burn your tongue. *Never use rubbing alcohol or wood alcohol for internal use* — these are extremely toxic if ingested! You can use rubbing alcohol to make an herbal liniment for external use, but personally I like good old vodka for this as well. Yes, it is more expensive, but it's safer. Decant your tinctures into little dropper bottles, which can be purchased from or ordered through your local pharmacy. Naturally, label all your herbal products as to date, contents, and use.

Herbal Wine

Certain herbs can be steeped in wine—consider May wine, in which sweet woodruff is steeped in German white wine—but these are for a more immediate consumption, as they do not store very long. They can be considered a pleasant way to take your medicine or a medicinal way to take your pleasure—you decide.

To infuse wine with herbs, pour one bottle (1 fifth, or ⅘ quart, or 750 ml) of wine into a quart jar, into which you have placed a half cup fresh, clean herbs or edible flowers, the combination of which your imagination is the only limit. If you are using dried spices such as clove or cinnamon, just add a few pieces, as they are quite pungent.

One example of herb-infused wine for remedial use is called the elder rob, which is dried elderberries with a cinnamon stick mulled in a dry red wine such as burgundy. Of course, infusing herbs in wine primarily for their flavorful effects is completely permissible. See page 208, "M is for Mint," for a refreshing example of a flowery herb-flavored wine.

Oil Extracts

You can steep certain herbs in oil to make healing rubs for many purposes. Pure olive oil has a good shelf life and is the most common oil used for salves; almond oil is nice base for special body oils.

HERB-INFUSED OIL—In a small saucepan, place one pint of oil and two ounces dried plant material or four ounces fresh herbs, using more oil if necessary to cover. Put the saucepan on the barest flicker of heat and steep the herbs in the oil for several hours, stirring occasionally; make sure it doesn't scorch. Depending on the plant material, you may want to steep for a couple days; in this case, you would turn the heat off overnight (cover with a towel so it can still evaporate) and start the gentle heat again in the morning. The oil is ready when it smells fragrant and has a deep color from the herbs—in fact, the herbs will have lost some of their own green color. Strain to remove the herbs and wait for the oil to cool somewhat before storing in a clean, dry bottle.

I have found that a mini slow cooker is an excellent gentle warming vessel for steeping herbs in oil, especially fresh herbs, because you can leave the lid off so the water in the plant material can evaporate and you can keep it going for a couple days without any worry. If you don't use some sort of heat and merely soak fresh herbs and oil in a jar with the lid on, the herbs will mold—yuk! Food safety advisory: for this reason, it is no longer recommended to infuse garlic in oil for any length of time unless vinegar is involved, otherwise it can grow botulism in an anaerobic (airless) environment. I realize you won't likely be consuming your herbal oil extracts, but the same principle is involved. Therefore, if you're using fresh herbs, I recommend a gentle heat of some type. Oil extracts of herbs such as birch twigs or cottonwood buds make an excellent analgesic rub and smell fabulous. Use St. John's wort oil for bruises and muscle spasms. You can steep fragrant flower petals and herbs for an after-shower body oil. Store your oils in glass bottles. Oil extracts are not the same as essential oils, which are a concentrated distilled product rather than plant parts steeped in a carrier oil as above. You will need to make herbal oil extracts in order to make the following remedies.

Herbal Salves, Ointments, Balms, and Unguents

What do you give a pig with a sore throat? *Oinkment!*

Anyway…these interchangeable terms refer to remedies used for healing superficial scrapes and abrasions and various skin ailments. They are oil extracts prepared as above, then thickened or hardened with beeswax or some other sort of solid fat such as cocoa butter, coconut oil, or if you have a hunter in the house, rendered deer's tallow. Lip balm is a glorified salve. Make the salve using herbs according to your particular need; for example, you can use cedar leaves as an antifungal, chickweed and plantain as an emollient, Oregon grape root to prevent infection, or comfrey root for quick healing.

BASIC SALVE RECIPE—To one pint warm oil extract prepared as instructed above, stir in approximately one ounce grated beeswax. If you're using another type of thickener, you will have to experiment, because it's hard to estimate how viscous the oil will be. To check for hardness, scoop up a teaspoon of the oil-wax blend and pour it onto a small plate; after a few minutes, it will have cooled, and you can test its consistency then. If it's too soft, it will slosh around in the container; if it's too hard, it will be difficult to get a swipe out of it. Salves can be compounded with more than one type of oil extract or an oil extract made of several different herbs. You can also add small amounts of other ingredients as well, such as honey, lanolin, or vitamin E oil. Be sure to label and date. Store your salves in small, wide-mouthed jars, but do not cover until the salve is cool. Find pretty jars for gift giving.

Making salves is definitely an organic, experiential process and sometimes a little messy, but that really is part of the fun. Children can take part in the project by helping identify and harvest the healing plants. See page 145, "G is for Grandma's Magic Healing Salve," for a further exploration of children and herbs, and page 215, "M is for Mother's Tummy Rub," for a salve that smells good enough to eat.

LIP BALM—Similar to salves, make the oil extract with one cup almond oil and one-fourth cup dried rose petals or calendula petals (or both); steep for several hours to overnight, and remember to use very gentle heat. Strain and return to heating vessel, then add approximately one tablespoon grated beeswax, stirring with a chopstick to blend. You can also add up to a teaspoon of vitamin E oil and a dab of honey or cocoa butter, or try a drop or two of glycerin-based vanilla or almond flavoring (not to be confused with the alcohol-based vanilla extract you might be used to). Blend thoroughly, and then carefully pour into several small containers convenient for dipping a pinky finger into, and be sure to leave the lids off until completely cool. Homemade lip balm makes an excellent gift.

Herbal Syrups and Elixirs

Use herbal syrups as a remedy for sore throats and coughs, and for tonics made with bitter herbs. Rosehips, elderberries, blackberries, violet leaf and flower, and red clover blossom all make good syrups, as does the infamous horehound. Of course, some of these herbal syrups are good to use on foods such as pancakes, hot cereal, glazing on roast meat, or hot drinks. I sometimes use honey to make my herbal syrups, which is soothing in and of itself for a sore throat, especially with a little squeeze of lemon. Please note that infants under one year old should not be fed honey, as it can carry botulism spores that are harmless to adults but can be harmful to the baby. One stirring-teaspoon of syrup is the usual dose for an "average-sized" adult; use more for bigger folks, less for little ones. Up to eight doses per day may be safely ingested.

BASIC HERBAL SYRUP — In a small saucepan, boil one quart water with two ounces dried or four ounces fresh plant material; turn down the heat and simmer uncovered until reduced by half, leaving one pint, about twenty minutes. Strain, then add a half cup honey, stirring until blended. If using sugar rather than honey, use one cup sugar and, when adding to the strained herbal decoction, return to medium heat until it's well dissolved before decanting, just a couple minutes. Pour the hot liquid into sterilized bottles, label, and date. The syrup should be refrigerated and will keep about three months.

Ways to use herbal syrups include elderberry elixir to chase off flu symptoms; comfrey root, mullein leaf, and hawthorn berries for a soothing expectorant; or violet flower syrup added to hot water for a delicate tea. Rosehip syrup is very interesting, almost applelike. Imagine a variety of minted syrups. Decanting into decorative bottles makes a beautiful gift presentation for culinary syrups.

Satisfying Work

The recipes and techniques described above are not meant to replace competent medical care when that becomes necessary, but for common colds, minor injuries, and so on, Grandma's ways were and still are often the best ways. Crafting a kitchen apothecary is one way to get in touch with how it was done before life became accelerated and specialized, when we still knew where things came from. I suggest you keep notes of your work. Plant some herbs in a patio pot for your concoctions. Don't be afraid to experiment within the guidelines. And, most importantly, have fun!

Why Local Herbs?

I would like to ramble on a bit about why I recommend local herbs for home remedies and healing medicine. By "herbs," I mean wild and domestic plants that can be used on or in the body for remedial or culinary use. By "local," I mean around your home or somewhere in the nearby vicinity or generalized region, wherever that may be at the time. I will also give mention to a few non-local but very useful common items that I think are worth keeping around for home remedies.

They're Economical

One reason I recommend this approach is the cost. If you learn to identify wild healing plants, your cost is minimal:

- a basket in which to collect herbs (heck, you could even use a brown paper bag)
- a pocket knife, which you probably already have and will last for years
- a good field guide, which may cost up to $25 but is also a lifelong investment

After these initial investments, the herbs you harvest become the gifts you receive for your efforts. I realize that you have to collect the herbs in spring and summer in order to use them in winter, but this will give you something to think about in the meantime. Read the section "Harvesting Herbs—and Then What?" on page 21 for thoughts on how and when to go about gathering and the kind of attitude involved in this giving-and-receiving approach.

If you want to grow your own herbs, you will still need the basket and knife or pruners, but you'll want to look at a gardening guide for the how-to's. Also, local plant nurseries usually have a very informative staff who are willing and able to share their knowledge and excitement for growing things with customers in need.

They're Everywhere

Now, you may think you don't know where to begin your search for wild medicinals. But maybe you like to hike or bike, or say your friend lives on a farm or ranch with acres to roam. Or maybe you yourself live rurally; healing plants wait right outside your door. You've probably already seen some of them. Some people pull 'em out as weeds in their garden. Believe me, I have pulled out more than my share of chickweed, although this is later in the summer when it actually does become a prolific pest, but I eat the early spring growth of this tasty, common "weed." Even town-dwellers have "wild medicinals" such as plantain growing around the yard; all you have to do is look. Inquiring minds want to know.

Choosing Your Site

If you know the land you wish to forage from hasn't been sprayed with chemicals, there's a good starting point. If it's someone else's land, get permission first. As for cultivated healing plants, your only limits are space and the environmental requirements of a given plant. In regard to what herbs to grow for medicines, you can buy starts from your local garden center (I suggest a privately owned one over a mega-mart) or through mail order. Starts are often better than seeds for perennials, as certain varieties do not grow true from seed. Much more fun and congenial is to get starts from friends and neighbors who are thinning their herb beds in the spring. After all, you'll be thinning your herb bed in a few years too and so can return the favor. Growing your own herbs—or anything else, for that matter—will stimulate natural wellness and healing for the body, mind, and spirit, whether through quiet contemplation or eager-beaver activity. Balance is achieved because gardening involves both. Harvesting from the wild is also holistically beneficial, and you get to see things you wouldn't ordinarily, such as little spotted fawns or spotted fawn lilies. It's all a part of what I call natural magic.

They're Convenient

Another reason to use local herbs is that they're always there, though not necessarily at any time of year—that's part of the planning-for-winter stuff I mentioned above, with you traipsing about the countryside gathering goldenrod and yarrow and elderflowers, drying them, and storing them away for the flu you hope you don't get. If you know how to recognize the wild plants at home, you'll be able to identify them in your travels away from home later. I recall a trip to Southern California some years ago to see our grandkids, and part of the journey took us over some pretty high terrain, specifically Smokey Bear Flats, over 9,000 feet in elevation. As we were walking our lively Siberian husky, we came across some miniature yarrow plants barely three inches tall, much shorter than the plants at home, which average at least a foot. Also growing amongst the yarrow and sprawling junipers were teeny-tiny violets, except their leaves were somewhat fuzzy like an African violet instead of smooth as they are at home; I reasoned that because it was such a dry environment, they grew little hairs in order to gather any and all moisture they could from the atmosphere. What a phenomenal discovery! So you see, getting to know the wild plants in your neck of the woods could lead to exciting discoveries when you journey elsewhere, comparing one species with another. Now, that's my kind of fun!

Say Hello in There

When you use local herbs, you are using the tried and true remedies of your grandmothers. I remember my own Gramma Lil talking about plantain leaf, that her folks used it on scrapes and bruises. Who knew? I kicked myself for not asking her more, sooner. Take some time and talk to the old ones. Ask them what simples their folks used for coughs, colds, and other common ailments. (I have heard of people using kerosene for all sorts of conditions, a remedy I think I'll avoid.) I spoke with a young man a while back who mentioned the onion-syrup remedy for coughs; I was surprised to learn that this "kid" knew about a natural remedy, which he learned from his folks, of course. People are usually quite willing to share this kind of information, especially when they see that others are interested in natural healing too. So don't shy away from asking.

Some Non-Local Items

There a few items that are difficult to make or grow that aren't exactly local but are very worthwhile having on hand. I'll tell you what and why.

Capsicum, or cayenne pepper, is often grown in the home garden, but it's not always easy to get them to ripen here in northern Idaho. So I buy it in bulk powdered form, and from there capsule it up as needed. As a healing plant, cayenne acts as a catalyst and is often used to "kick start" other herbs into action through the circulatory system by opening the capillaries. Cayenne is warming to the body and is tonic to the stomach and intestines, which is very important during illness. I may as well add ginger root to this list. Ginger's action is similar to cayenne; it gets the other herbs activated once they're already in the system.

Another non-local item I use is sea salt. Now salt, in and of itself, is not harmful. Salt is a crystal, as we all know, and very powerful. Excessive use of salt (and processed foods) can be detrimental, as anyone with high blood pressure knows. Some body types require more salt, and in the summer, many mineral salts besides sodium are depleted through perspiration. This long-sought-after commodity is something we use and need every day. Some herbs, such as alfalfa and nettles, and the sea vegetables can replace salt and are very high in other valuable minerals. You can even use sea salt in the bath (see "B is for Bathing Beautiful," page 70).

I also buy apple cider vinegar, the organic health food store kind. This vinegar is a concentrated food and medicine for which there are many healthful uses. It is a stimulant, an astringent, has a cooling effect on the skin, and is antiseptic to some microorganisms. It contains most of the minerals that fresh apples do, including potassium. The pectin in apple cider vinegar has absorbing qualities in the intestines that aid in the elimination of certain viruses; this is of special benefit during the cold and flu season. Cider vinegar can be made at home, but it is easier to buy. I think it's important to keep plenty of it around because so many remedies are based on this simple food staple. I have provided many examples of ways to use vinegar in its very own chapter (see "V is for Vinegar," page 277).

Then there are cooking spices such as clove and cinnamon that do not grow even remotely nearby, and my favorite frankincense and myrrh that I burn (or, rather, melt) on the wood stove, but these are somewhat incidental to the above-mentioned items.

Keep It Local, Keep It Simple

All in all, I believe you will have fun getting to know the plants in your yard, your neighborhood, and your region. Getting out in the fresh air and sunshine won't hurt you either, and you may, in fact, discover other things you weren't expecting along the way ... but I don't want to give away all the surprises before you get the chance to find them yourself.

Harvesting Herbs — and Then What?

Many people have asked me when the best time is to harvest herbs. I tell them that it depends on what part of the plant you need. Root, leaf, flower, seed, bark, and fruit are each harvested at different times of the year, as well as different times of the day. And besides wanting to know when to harvest herbs, folks also want to know what to do with them once they're harvested. There are several different ways to process and store them.

The following is what I've learned from other books, through personal experience, and from my own intuition. I have used many methods over the years, some of which I've streamlined and some of which I've expanded upon.

First Things First

Naturally, you want to select plants that are free of sprays and auto emissions; I can't stress this often enough. Dust isn't exactly desirable either. (I'm assuming your garden plants won't have any of these issues.) In addition, if harvesting from the wild, you should leave at least half of the plants intact, unharvested, in order for them to replenish themselves for the following years. A few years ago, I learned about the life cycle of a local plant, *Lomatium dissectum*, the root of which we dig and tincture for lung congestion, very powerful and used in small quantities. Well, I found out that some of the larger roots could be up to forty years old! So we restricted how often we harvest (every few years) and from where (several different stands) so we don't deplete the local population. Oh yeah, and we talk to the plant first before harvesting. No, I'm not kidding. My own personal ritual is to say a prayer of thanks to the spirit of the plant for giving itself to us. I also leave some sort of offering, a snippet of hair maybe, or even a bit of natural fertilizer if appropriate. This is where intuition comes into play; don't be afraid to use yours. What do you think the plant would appreciate?

I'd like to add here that these methods are for harvesting wild herbs for your own personal use, not for selling commercially. If that's what you're into, I suggest you check with your local ranger district and see what rules and regulations apply to the commercial harvest of forest and range plants. I've seen a lot of abuse over the years in the form of erosion and the destruction of plants and native grasses from people driving their ATVs where they don't belong, picking berries and mushrooms for money. Most of these folks are not harvesting with any heartfelt commitment to preserving nature or anything else. You might want to get in touch with renowned herbalist Rosemary Gladstar and her organization United Plant Savers for more information about the ecological and ethical harvesting of wild plants for commercial use. Another good resource to learn about ecologically sound harvesting methods is Gregory L. Tilford's *The EcoHerbalist's Fieldbook: Wildcrafting in the Mountain West*, which focuses on wild plants of the western United States.

Roots and Other Underground Parts

When you harvest a root, you are taking the whole plant, which means it won't grow back. The exceptions to this are plants such as wild ginger, in which case the "root" is actually a rhizome, or underground stem, and whatever breaks off usually grows back, especially if the root crown is replanted; Oregon grape root is another such example. A plant such as dandelion, however, will be taken whole. Most people aren't worried about depleting the dandelion population, though, or burdock, bramble, or comfrey, for that matter. Truth be told, I have yet to see comfrey die out, even after being inadvertently rototilled with the rest of the garden—it just makes more comfrey plants.

So, when do you dig up roots anyway? Either early spring or late fall, and early in the morning. The reason? Plants have periods of rest, and when they are resting, the root is the most energized part of the plant. Early spring and early morning, the plant is just beginning to awaken, and the carbohydrate is still in storage (the root is the storage center of the plant). In the fall, part of the summer's growth has gone back to feed the root in order to continue the cycle and come back the following year. If you harvest in mid-summer, for example, you'll get a root that is less potent, because the plant is more interested in ripening seeds then. One advantage to fall harvesting is that you've been able to locate the desired plant(s) by identifying its more obvious parts, i.e., the flowers and leaves, and maybe visiting it a few times to let it know your intentions—sort of like a new puppy. You could also make note of the plant's location in the fall with a ribbon or something and go back to it again in the spring, when its "juices" will be fresh and clear.

Leaves

The leaf of a plant is an energetic "receiver." There is a magical process called photosynthesis, whereby the leaves, via the green substance called chlorophyll, manufacture food using energy from the sun: they miraculously synthesize carbohydrates for the plant from carbon dioxide (in the air) and water, putting pure oxygen back into the air. Even houseplants add oxygen to a home; the more the merrier (though I actually know someone who can kill an air fern, but I won't mention any names). Because the leaves receive most of their energy during full sunlight, you should harvest them midday and as near as possible to when the flower is in bloom.

Flowers

At peak florescence, or flowering, the visible parts of a plant (including the leaves) are at full potency, and it practically vibrates with energy; if you watch long enough, you can just about see it breathe. So, again, midday is the best time to harvest flowers, when they are stretching their fullest to the sun. Just before all the flowers have opened is best too, because as the flowers fade, the energy goes toward reproduction, or seed making, and the potency is reduced. For example, cutting stalks of mint just as the flowers bloom is ideal because both the leaf and flower are at optimum potency. If you are harvesting individual flower heads, such as red clover or violet, these should be taken when fully open, when their fragrance is most intense; in the case of roses, take only the petals and not the seedpod, otherwise you'll take autumn's rosehips.

Fruits (Which Are Technically Plant Ovaries)

Speaking of rosehips, or elderberries or hawthorn berries, these should be picked when just becoming perfectly ripe, not overripe. You don't want them turning into wine in your drying basket or food dehydrator ... or do you? If you are going to use them fresh, as in a tincture (or even in pies or jams), fully ripe is good, but if you are going to dry and store them, you don't want them too squishy. Some people say these fruits taste best after a light frost, which is true for pleasurable eating, but I think they dry and store better if harvested before that point. Be sure to give them plenty of air circulation when drying to avoid any mold from forming.

Seeds

If you wait to harvest the seed until it's completely mature, it may have lost some of its potency. The seed is the life-center of a plant, the germ for the next generation. An overripened seed, while certainly not dead, is not as energized as a just-on-the-verge-of-ripening seed. This is important in aromatic culinary seeds such as dill or fennel; harvest the seed heads midday, before the seeds are ready to fall off—in other words, slightly underripe. They will fully ripen after being harvested if left on the head; tie the stems in bunches and hang them upside down, perhaps with a brown paper bag loosely tied around the actual heads to catch any falling seeds and to keep the dust off. These culinary seeds are remedial as well (see "S is for Spice Rack Remedies," page 255). Their aromatic quality contributes to their potency; therefore, you want to catch them at their peak.

Bark (and I Don't Mean "Woof"!)

I don't often harvest tree bark, but should you desire to do so, springtime is best, when the sap is fresh and running. Remove a small branch from the tree with a saw or sharp loppers. Then remove the whole bark with a hefty knife, and scrape off and keep the fleshy inner bark, which is the medicinal substance and is often red, pink, or orange, from the rough outer bark. This may actually take some doing, but be patient. Do not take any bark from the main trunk, for, unless you plan to cut it down for whatever reason, this will damage or even kill the tree—bad karma! Check out page 299, "X is for Xylem & Phloem," to learn more about the inner workings of tree bark.

Now What?

So there you are with some nice bunches of mint, a quart of St. John's wort flowers, a basket of rosehips, several strands of Oregon grape root, wondering what to do next. Again, that depends on what part of the plant you've gathered.

In Bunches

In the case of stemmy plants like alfalfa, mint, yarrow, oregano, and so on, the simplest and most effective way is to tie them up in small bunches or bind the stem ends with a rubber band (which works well as the herbs dry because of the stretch factor) and hang them in a dry, dust-free, semi-dark place. Hang them from the rafters, suspended wire or clothesline, or a wooden clothes-drying rack. Even decorative flower arrangements can be gathered in bunches and dried this way.

On Screens

You can use recycled screen panels (well washed and dried) or buy or make new ones to dry herbs. You can prop the screen up between two chairs or balance them on the rungs of the above-mentioned clothes-drying rack. This method works well for large, thick, or heavy plant matter, such as split and quartered roots, dill weed fronds, large mullein leaves, or even calendula flowers. Spread out the herbs evenly so they don't touch and so there is plenty of air circulation between them. An oscillating fan is a useful but not necessary piece of equipment you can use to add air movement to the situation. In fact, air circulation is the most important factor in drying herbs, much more so than heat, which, if excessive, can compromise the potency of the herbs.

A Tisket, a Tasket

You can dry 'em in a basket. Take flowers such as red clover, chamomile, or marigolds, and fruits such as rosehips and hawthorn berries, and spread them in large, shallow baskets. Make sure you toss them around at least once a day for that all-important air circulation. In my experience, rosehips dry better if you split them open using a sharp paring knife; you can cut them in half, or if they're huge, such as from the *Rosa rugosa* variety, into quarters; there will be small yellow seeds inside — dry these too, along with the fruit. Sometimes roots are dried in baskets as well.

Not On My Watch

I hear that some folks nuke their herbs and dry them in a micro-wave oven. Please, please, please! After all the kindness you have shown the plants, after all the effort you have taken to be gentle on the earth, don't dry your herbs this way! While this method most certainly quick-dries the herb, it destroys all the life force of it, which definitely alters their healing properties. No, I don't have a microwave oven in my home; I don't even have a cell phone.

What About Freshly Harvested Herbs?

If you don't want to dry your wild or domestic healing plants, I refer you to the Kitchen Apothecary section on page 3 for a multitude of ways to process them into useful homemade concoctions such as syr-ups, oils, and salves. These are a lot of fun to make, and your friends and family will be grateful that you took the time and energy to pro-duce products to soothe their symptoms as well as their souls.

Trust Yourself

As for the culinary herbs (and some of these do double-duty, as I have pointed out), here's another chance to use your intuition. Just what *will* you do with all those elderberries, now that you have a gallon of them? Jam, pie, homemade wine …?

The Pantry

It's late October, and I just spent the last few days reorganizing my pantry. There are seven shelves (including the floor), each about nine feet long, and it was looking like a fire sale before a hurricane. With the tomato windfall from the garden this year, there's a whole shelf with just tomato products. It's a food bank almost, and there's something in me that thinks food is more valuable than money. I highly recommend keeping as well-stocked a pantry as your finances will allow; buy organic if you can. It should be obvious that I like to cook and putter in the kitchen, and while my philosophy is to choose local ingredients first, there's no harm in exploring your culinary fantasies either. What follows are some things I have realized about food over the years, and I share this with you in the spirit of fun and what works for me.

Spice It Up

With the variety of herbs and spices alone—which are available locally, at farmer's markets, or through mail order—you can turn an ordinary pan of noodles into a culinary romp across the continents. So there's a good place to start your pantry—the herb and spice cabinet. Get a small amount of all the kinds you can find. I urge you to check out recipe books from the library or search the Internet for regional, international, and ethnic cuisine—whatever suits your fancy. If you're like me, you'll have a blast getting a taste for the flavors and nuances of a culture, learning the geography and the history, even trying to learn a few words in the appropriate language. A gentle reminder here: use a light hand with any new flavors you initially experiment with. I speak from experience as one who tried to invent a quasi-African stew with yams and peanuts and—let's not go there just now!

About Oil

I use extra-virgin olive oil for all sorts of cooking. I know most chez's recommend pure olive oil for the softer flavor, but this is what I prefer—and you should do what you prefer. I also use sunflower oil for its mild, unimposing flavor. I use plain, untoasted sesame oil in some of the Asian-inspired dishes I prepare, especially fried rice. For salads I use EVOO or occasionally hazelnut oil—yummy! I sometimes use a fantastically corny-tasting unrefined corn oil when fixing corn bread. Buy quality over quantity—most oils do not keep for long. I don't use margarine at all; I fry my eggs in butter, thank you, and also spread it on the toast. I have never used ghee—clarified butter used in East Indian cooking—but I understand that it stores well. For baking, I use butter or oil, and in pastry crust, I use butter. All right, I know that butter is saturated fat, but at least it's real, and we're talking pastry, not stir fry. Just don't eat it all the time. I personally cannot abide by hydrogenated vegetable shortening.

Vinegar, or What Do You Call a Cat Who Drinks Lemonade?

I keep white wine vinegar in my pantry; it's used for salad dressings on occasion, but I use it most often for canning pickled vegetables such as asparagus and green beans. I also keep apple cider vinegar (for therapeutic and cosmetic use also), balsamic vinegar, and fruit- and herb-flavored vinegars in stock. I seldom use plain white vinegar except for washing or cleaning something. See page 277, "V is for Vinegar," for information on how to make these flavored vinegars.

Relish the Idea

As for commercially bottled sauces and condiments, there's a wide world of them out there, and these are what I like to keep around: natural soy sauce (did you know there are brands that don't actually have any "soy sauce" in them? Read the label!); oyster sauce and fish sauce (and yes, there actually is oyster and fish in these); health food store mayo; grainy and Dijon mustard; wasabi powder; Worcestershire sauce and Tabasco sauce; pimientos, anchovies, capers, and olives; ketchup and sweet relish; and so on. I recently discovered brined green peppercorns—whoa! Also included in this list could be nut butters and jams and pickles and such.

About Salt

It seems most people prefer sea salt, although I do wonder about the purity of the sea these days. There are several specialty salts available, but as a table salt, the one I prefer is totally unrefined, speckled from other minerals, and unfortunately very expensive. I use plain, non-iodized sea salt for canning. Kosher salt is wonderful sprinkled on salads and baked goods for both the pureness of flavor and its wonderful texture; I recommend Diamond Crystal brand because there are no additives. If you cannot tolerate salt, I suggest you learn how to use herbs and spices to flavor your food, although salt definitely brings out all the other flavors. Canning vegetables without salt is a mistake, in my opinion; they taste hideously flat.

Sweetie Pie

I rarely use white sugar; to me, it's akin to "the cocaine of sugar-cane." However, compared to high-fructose corn syrup (a genetically modified substance), sugar (sucrose that is) seems the lesser of the evils. However, just like politics, evil is still evil, and I know I'm not kidding myself when I use organic dried cane juice; sugar by any other name is still sugar, even if it's groovy sugar. Once consumed, honey is assimilated in the body just like sugar, even though you use less; molasses is sugar "tar," but it sure makes a good Q sauce (see page 237); and don't even talk to me about fructose (another white crystalline substance) — I'll get mine straight from the fruit, thank you very much. Date sugar (which is ground, dried dates, a complex carbohydrate compared to plain sugar) is wonderful in desserts such as apple crisp. Malted barley or rice syrup is tasty, even if the flavor may not be what you expect from "sweet." Maple syrup adds a rich, deep flavor to carob brownies. Sorghum syrup makes awesome caramel corn. Here's a tasty way to use honey: gently melt it to make fruit-, herb- or spice-infused syrups (see page 3, the Kitchen Apothecary section, for how-to). It's difficult to resist real pastry from the local bakery (at least it is for me), so my advice on sweets is Excess in Moderation. Learn to satisfy your sweet tooth with less, and taste the real food. When I use a dessert recipe from a "conventional" cookbook, I almost always reduce the amount of sugar called for by at least a third.

The Baker's Dozen

For most baking, the basics are all you really need: baking powder and baking soda; cream of tartar; dry baking yeast; cocoa and carob powder; chocolate and carob chips; extracts and flavorings such as vanilla, almond, and lemon; instant tapioca for thickening fruit pies. I use whole wheat pastry flour for most dessert baking, and unbleached flour and hard red whole wheat flour for breads. Buy variety flours, such as rye, millet, or barley, in small quantities to insure freshness. Keep them in a cool, dry place, preferably in glass jars.

Beans and Grains

Dried beans and whole grains, once prepared, are as fancy or as plain as you like, but all are delicious and nutritious. Stored in glass jars or canisters on your pantry shelf or even on your countertop, they are a kaleidoscope of variety. If you buy them in large quantities, remember that they do not keep much longer than a year or two at most; otherwise the beans will get drier—if you can imagine—and be hard to reconstitute completely, and with too long of storage, some grains will go rancid. Most beans and legumes need to be soaked several hours before cooking. Most whole grains take at least half an hour to cook. Consider the convenience of rolled whole grains such as oats, barley, corn, and rye. Rolled oats are usually a given in most pantries, but the others are a nice addition to baked goods. I sometimes like to add rolled rye to pizza dough, and rolled barley is a hearty change from cooked oatmeal.

There are quite a few good books dealing specifically with grain and bean cookery, in all their glory. If you are vegetarian, you must educate yourself about these foods, which are literally the backbone of your diet; the combination of beans and grains make a complete protein that they by themselves do not. Tofu may be a decent low-fat protein source, but it is a processed food, while beans and grains are whole foods. I find the history of these foods fascinating, as they are the agricultural and cultural building blocks of most civilizations. Who would have imagined a sweet bean paste for desserts, or buckwheat and onion stuffed inside a dumpling skin? The endless variety of grain-bean dishes deserves more than a cursory exploration. I can only hope that the genetic experimentation on these basic crops won't mess things up beyond recognition.

My Friends Are Nutty ... and Seedy

And I love them for it! What a fascinating variety they are, too. Nuts and seeds are a good source of protein and healthy fat, as long as they are fresh. Keep small quantities of nuts in a cool place, perhaps your refrigerator. Almonds, soaked overnight in plenty of water and then drained, are a crunchy, plump surprise. I use sunflower seeds in everything from granola to quesadillas. I'm still waiting for my hazelnut bushes to produce, so until then, I buy them in the fall and enjoy them in shortbread, pilaf, and risotto. Pistachios are great—do you remember the red-dyed variety when you were a kid, when you could easily tell who snacked on what the night before?

Yes, We Can

As far as canned foods go, my choices are simple: whole green chilies, and lots of 'em. Oh yeah, and baby corn. I also live on a Mexican-style hot tomato sauce in a yellow can with a duck on it (El Pato Salsa de Chili Fresco)—it's hot, it's addictive, and in our house, it's purchased by the case. No, it's not organic, but nothing else comes close in taste, except for last year's home-canned golden cha-cha sauce (which was actually better), but we go through the homemade stuff pretty fast. I also keep in stock canned beans like kidney and pinto and cannellini, and fruits like pineapple. I buy apple juice by the case for making smoothies if I don't have any preserved. I love to do my own canning of garden fruits and veggies, but I realize this isn't for everyone.

Use Your Noodle

The infinite variety of dried Italian-type pastas and Asian noodles ought to keep you eating for weeks. Some fresh types can be frozen, such as wonton and Chinese wheat noodles. I won't instruct you here as to what noodle goes with what sauce or seasoning; just study your choice of cuisine and let your imagination fly. Your only mistake will be not trying.

Brrr-r-r-r!

One item I always keep in my freezer (besides meat) is chicken and buffalo broth, in pints and quarts. (The yearly buffalo run is a whole story unto itself.) I try to freeze up broccoli and spinach from my garden too, if I've planned ahead and can keep the deer out. And now that the blueberry bushes have really kicked in, we freeze some of these, along with raspberries, for pies and smoothies. If you can't grow your own, find your local farmer's market, get to know the vendors, and see if you can buy in quantity. Berries are very easy to freeze: carefully tumble the berries onto a waxed paper–lined baking sheet in a single layer, and place in the freezer (I do not recommend washing berries first unless they are very dusty); a few hours later, place the frozen berries into a freezer bag or container. Better toss a couple in your mouth while you're at it—kids of all ages love frozen berry pops! If it's veggies you want to freeze, they'll have to be blanched first. Get a chart and instruction booklet from your County Extension office as to the timing and so forth (or see page 36 for more food-preservation resources).

Fresh!

My basic produce basket, especially during the cold months, holds garlic, potatoes, onions, garlic, shallots, carrots, cabbage, garlic, lemons, cilantro, garlic, bananas, apples, romaine, garlic, cauliflower, and hot peppers. Did I mention garlic? Most fresh fruit from the grocery store tastes like crap to me, so I hardly ever eat it. Naturally, there's a lot more variety during the farmer's market and home-gardening season.

Cheese It

When I buy and use dairy products, including eggs, the majority are from organically produced sources; I don't want any growth hormones in my food, thankyouverymuch. (I really don't care if it's certified either.) Some of the imported European cheeses usually aren't labeled as such, but I think you have to weigh the quantity and frequency of consumption against the urging of your taste buds to just go with it ... so, let your taste buds have their say once in a while.

If We Weren't Supposed to Eat Animals ...

...then why did God make them out of meat?

Yes, I cook meat and eat it. I also harvest and butcher and brine and smoke and sausage and even jerk it on occasion. My first choice is always wild, whether mammal, bird, or fish; next is home or locally raised. Now, I could get onto a very tall soapbox here concerning a number of issues, including the ethics of eating meat, religion, cultural traditions, despicable farming practices, hunting for sport instead of for food, current government standards and/or the lack thereof, people who think they have the answers for everyone else... but I digress. If you can't or don't or won't eat meat, simply avoid those recipes in this book that include it (and there are only a few) or substitute your preference. As far as I'm concerned, a freshly harvested carrot is just as sentient as any of the walkers and squawkers, and yogurt is still alive and kicking when you eat it. I do not propose to set into stone any particular philosophy except Gratitude for the food in my larder and Awareness of the sources from whence they came. Personally, I have never been able to understand the whole "fake meat" thing.

Is She Finished Yet?

To summarize the pantry and its contents, I strive to use whole and minimally processed foods as much as possible. I am very eclectic in my diet and my approach to cooking, and I do not dwell too much on any particular regimen except for wanting good, whole, organically grown food. Support your local growers and producers if you can't do it yourself. I am blessed by my involvement with a food co-op, which definitely helps offset the higher cost of quality bulk foods; I'll bet there's one in your neighborhood too.

Have fun stocking your pantry. Take pleasure in imagining the wonderful dishes you'll create with a bit of this and a dash of that. Just don't try to stock it all at once—you might not have any cash left for, let's say, cookbooks!

Handbooks and References I Reach For Most Often

You might notice that I have gone into great detail describing certain steps in these recipes and remedies. This is to assure success in your creations and to assure your safety. The instructions for making herbal vinegar are a case in point: I *re-e-e-ally* want it to come out right for you.

As author of this book, as a hands-on herbalist, as a mother and grandma, and as a certified Master Food Preserver/Food Safety Advisor, I feel a personal responsibility to present correct information concerning herbs and wild plants and to explain the most current and generally-recognized-as-safe procedures for handling any food recipe in this book. However, since this is not an herb identification handbook or a food science text, nor am I a food scientist, I am somewhat limited in what can realistically be explained within the parameters of this book. So this chapter is devoted to some of those books, websites, and other resources I have used to get answers for my own questions. I want to help you learn to help yourself. This list does not endorse any particular authors or publications; it just so happens that I reach for these books and references more often than not.

Cookbooks I Have Used Over and Over Again

- *Cook's Illustrated* magazine
- *The Moosewood Cookbook* by Mollie Katzen
- *How to Bake* by Nick Malgieri
- *The Martha Stewart Living Cookbook*
- *The Seattle Times Cookbook*
- *The Passionate Palate* by Desirée Witkowski
- *The Kitchen Witch's Cookbook* by Patricia Telesco (includes recipes by yours truly)
- *Snackers* by Maureen & Jim Wallace
- *The Pioneer Lady's Country Kitchen* by Jane Watson Hopping

Some books that I just love to read include any book by Paula Wolfert. Some are visually stunning to look at, such as the herb cookbooks by author Emelie Tolley and photographer Chris Mead. I've had a baker's dozen of the Time/Life series *The Good Cook* for decades and refer to them often for the step-by-step photos of many techniques. If you can find old issues, look for *The Kitchen Garden* magazine by Taunton Press (these are the same folks who publish *Fine Woodworking* and *Fine Gardening* magazines); while no longer in print, it was a wonderful blend of creative cooking and kitchen gardening, with great photos. Another resource is, again, the Internet for a world wide web of recipes and cooking resources, such as Epicurious.com. I recommend scheduling a bit of time for this activity, as you can really get lost in the fun. Don't forget used book stores; they can be a great source of the obscure and unusual, which is the story of my life.

University/State Cooperative Extension Programs

These programs offer current canning and freezing procedures, backed by years of extensive research. Simply go online and search "[your state] Cooperative Extension," or ask at the library, or look in the phone book. These extension programs will be associated with at least one university in your state or a neighboring state, and some systems are multi-state. The Master Food Preservers and Master Gardeners are both programs of University Extension, but not all states or counties offer them. The National Center for Home Food Preservation is a program through the University of Georgia, and they offer a free course in learning how to preserve food; look for it online.

Books on Canning and Preserving (Be Sure to Reference with Extension Procedures)

- *Ball Blue Book Guide to Preserving* by Alltrista Corporation. They make the Ball and Kerr brand canning jars and lids, and update recipes regularly. This is the book your granny probably used, but please get a current

version. I found an ancient one at a yard sale that is so
out of date, it called for canning green beans in a water
bath canner for three hours—not recommended!

- *Well Preserved* by Mary Anne Dragan
- *Putting Food By* by Janet Greene & Ruth Hertzberg
- *Canning & Preserving Without Sugar* by Norma M. MacRae.
  I really like the options here, from honey to concentrated
  apple juice, for sweetening your home-grown products.
- *Stocking Up* by Rodale Press
- *Summer in a Jar* by Andrea Chessman. I like her recipes, but
  I do not recommend the procedure called "steam canning,"
  which is not recommended by Extension research.
- *So Easy to Preserve* by Cooperative Extension,
  the University of Georgia.
- Pomona's Universal Pectin, a two-part type of pectin,
  offers recipes with their product, which will gel with
  "any amount of any sweetener"—very versatile.
  This is the only type of pectin I have ever used.

Just like regular cookbooks, there are many canning cookbooks and websites as well as those mentioned on my list. If you find a recipe that leaves you unsure of the procedure, do not hesitate to contact your Cooperative Extension office; they will refer you to people like me, who will help you find the answers.

The next list alphabetically refers to books I have been reaching for since well before I became a grandma. While they are formally listed in the bibliography, I have annotated the more important texts that I have come to appreciate.

Books About Herbs and Wild Plants
for Food and Medicine

- *Herbal Medicine* and *The Complete Herbal Guide to Natural Health & Beauty* by Dian Dincin Buchman. The author gleaned some of these recipes from her Romanian grandmother, who learned from Gypsies.

- *Lewis Clark's Field Guide to Wildflowers of the Mountains in the Pacific Northwest* and *A Field Guide to Wildflowers of Forest and Woodland in the Pacific Northwest,* also by Lewis J. Clark. There are some good photos here.

- *Cunningham's Encyclopedia of Magical Herbs* by Scott Cunningham. The late, popular author has also written other magical encyclopedias, including aromatherapy and food, and obviously loved his subject matter.

- *Nature Bound Pocket Field Guide* by Ron Dawson. Very good photos.

- *Handbook of Edible Weeds* by James Duke. Duke is very knowledgeable, with years of experience with the USDA as well as personal experience. He has been leading indigenous plant tours of the Amazon and other places for years, with emphasis on preserving wild plant species.

- *Wild Roots* by Doug Elliot. A look at the unseen world.

- *Cornucopia — A Source Book of Edible Plants* by Stephen Facciola. This is one of the books I use for referencing the botanical names of plants. It is a veritable gold mine of plant types and sources to procure seed.

- *Weeds of Eastern Washington and Adjacent Areas* by Xerpha M. Gaines and D. G. Swan. Very good text on local plants (to me at least) and good drawings.

- *Stalking the Healthful Herbs* and *Stalking the Wild Asparagus* by Euell Gibbons. These are wonderful and informative narratives, never out of style.

- *Ethnobotany of Western Washington* by Erna Gunther

- *Montana: Native Plants and Early Peoples* by Jeff Hart. This book offers many anecdotal uses of plants, the author having interviewed many Native herbalists and elders in his research.

- *Wild Wildflowers of the West* by Edith S. Kinucan and Penny R. Brons. Edie was the person I sought out during the original *Wild & Weedy* publications to survey some of my articles for accuracy, and she has exposed a couple of urban legends more than once.

- *Common Herbs for Natural Health* by Juliette de Bairacli Levy. The author is a world traveler, and many of her remedies reflect this.

- *The Herb Book* by John Lust. A classic.

- *American Medical Ethnobotany: A Reference Dictionary* by Daniel E. Moerman. This book is unbelievable in its depth. Check out his extensive website at the University of Michigan, Dearborn.

- *Medicinal Plants of the Mountain West* and *Medicinal Plants of the Pacific West* by Michael Moore. These books are hands-down my favorite herbals. Moore is a very engaging writer and full of pertinent anecdotes.

- *Field Guide to Forest Plants of Northern Idaho* by Patricia Patterson, et al. This book is a USDA–Forest Service field guide, and I have used it for decades.

- *Discovering Wild Plants* by Janis J. Schofield. Good photos, useful entries.

- *Wild Teas, Coffees & Cordials: 60 Drinks of the Pacific Northwest* by Hilary Stewart. Beautiful drawings, interesting recipes.

- *The Ecoherbalist's Fieldbook* by Gregory L. Tilford. Similar to Moore's books in scope, Tilford's far-sighted vision concerns the sustainability of wildcrafting.
- *Northwest Wild Berries* by J. E. Underhill. How many do you recognize?
- *Healing Wise* by Susun Weed. Susun has written several other herbals; her approach is the Wise Woman tradition of healing—holistic and holy, and very useful and informative.
- *Earth Medicine Earth Food* by Michael A. Weiner. This book concerns the Native American use of many common plants.

This list is by no means complete. I have read and consulted (and purchased) literally hundreds of books over the years, which certainly doesn't take the place of actual fieldwork, but it's a start.

Of course, if you have any questions about the recipes or procedures in this book, or want to share any ideas or experiences, please do not hesitate to contact me via the publisher.

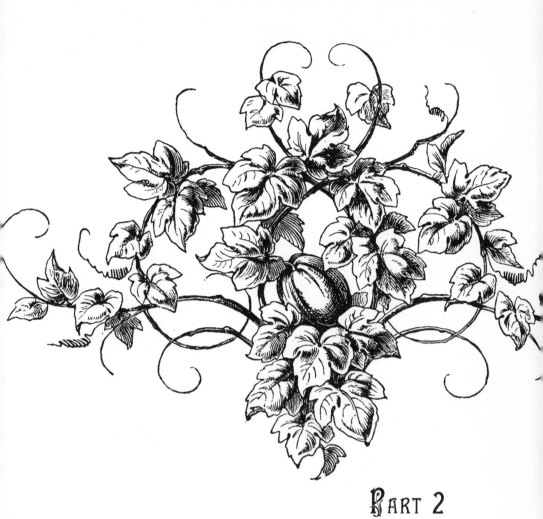

Part 2

Encyclopedia of
Recipes & Remedies

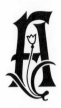

is for Alliums —
*the whole smelly,
delicious family*

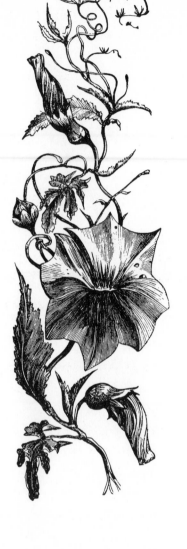

And it's a very unlikely plant family to be considered an aphrodisiac, if smell was the only thing you relied on for stimulation.

But wait, there's more! These luscious bulbs and leaves not only protect against vampires and absorb evil, they also repel aphids, and their bronze-colored skin makes one of the most popular dye plants. Eat freely of this aromatic family to prevent colds.

There's the venerable onion—red, white, and yellow—each with its multitude of form and variety; garlic, the stinking rose of culinary heaven, including the silver-skinned, rose-colored, and tawny; chives in the spring and garlic chives from China; scallions and spring onions to munch down whole; curious heirloom incarnations of the onion such as the top-setting, Egyptian, multiplier, potato, tree, and grandmother; and, naturally, the saucy shallot, without which there would be no French cuisine; and the aristocratic leek, emblem of Wales. Wild species of onion and garlic greet us with soft pink flowers and pungent leaves. Even the wild leek, or ramp, is cause for festive spring eating in the Appalachians and surrounding environs.

Gahlick, Dahling

The origin of onions and their ilk are uncertain, because they have been cultivated for so long. We do know that they have been used as food and medicine since prehistoric times. The sulfur compounds in these members of the lily family (yes, onions are a type of lily) are essential for many basic physiological functions. The juice from garlic is a known antifungal and antibiotic; you can rub a cut on your finger with fresh garlic, and while it will burn like the devil to do so, it will remain infection-free. Formed when garlic is crushed, the component called allicin is comparable to a 1 percent penicillin solution and is said to destroy *Candida albicans* as well as protect against amoebic dysentery (this doesn't mean if you contract dysentery, you should just eat garlic—you do need to get to a doctor). Garlic is also an antioxidant and helps reduce cholesterol. I refer you to "Z is for Zip" on page 310 for instructions on how to make a mighty garlic tonic to knock yer socks off.

Some folks make garlic tea when they feel a cold coming on, as a preventative. If their chest feels tight, they take a spoon of garlic syrup. I might add here that peeling garlic can be a bit of a chore, especially if your hands are wet. Once you get the cloves split apart from the head, I have found it helpful to trim off the stem end first (the part of the clove that attaches at the base) and then smack the individual clove open as directed below; it takes longer to explain it than to just do it. I have never found those tubular garlic peelers to be of any use. Do not use prepared garlic from a jar for these recipes.

. . . .

Garlic Tea

You will use a whole head of garlic for this recipe. To peel the garlic, lay each separated clove on a cutting board, then smack each one soundly by laying the side of a chef's knife on the clove and then hitting the side of the knife with your closed fist—watch out for the blade—then remove the peel. If you don't have a chef's knife, just use the heel of your hand and press down real hard until it pops. Next, toss the crushed cloves into a small saucepan with a quart of water and simmer until soft, about 20 minutes. Mash up the garlic in the broth with a fork, then strain. A pinch of sea salt for flavor doesn't hurt. Take half a cup every couple hours. This can be repeated the next day if you still have symptoms. Garlic tea will keep for a day or two refrigerated, but you might as well drink it till it's gone, in any case.

. . . .

Garlic Syrup

First, make garlic tea as instructed above, but let it steep overnight, unstrained. The next day, strain the tea, reheat until just warm, and add 4 tablespoons honey and 1 tablespoon apple cider vinegar; do not let the brew come to a boil. Take 1 or 2 tablespoons for adults, a teaspoon for children (but not babies), every hour or so, for two days. After that, refrigerate the syrup for up to a week or use it to baste chicken.

But garlic isn't an all-work-and-no-play kind of guy, oh, no. The entire city of Gilroy, California, devotes its livelihood to this most necessary of culinary basics. I have even heard of garlic ice cream, but that's where I draw the line. Oven roasting is one savory way to experience a kinder, gentler garlic. Spread it on toasted bread, pile it into mashed potatoes, or just squeeze it into your mouth when no one's looking (or even if they are).

. . . .

Roasted Garlic

Heat oven to 300 degrees. Lightly wipe a small glass oven dish or pie plate with olive oil. Remove most of the papery skin on a whole head of garlic without breaking up the head; repeat for however many heads you will be roasting. Then carefully slice off the very tip-top of the head, so that each clove is nicked open ever so slightly; this will make it easier to extrude the clove from its wrapper. For each head of garlic, mix 1 tablespoon olive oil and 1 tablespoon dry sherry or 1 teaspoon balsamic vinegar. Arrange garlic in baking dish, drizzle with the sherry-oil mixture, sprinkle with a little sea salt, then cover with foil or lid. Roast for about an hour or until very soft. Remove the cover for the last few minutes for the condensation to evaporate, but do not let the garlic burn or it will be bitter and ruined. After the garlic has cooled enough to touch, simply squeeze each softened clove into a small bowl for further use.

Unyum

A bit of sautéed onion is an excellent addition to homemade rye bread, and who isn't familiar with a chewy onion bagel? You can hollow out large yellow onions (first remove peel), stuff them with light bread crumbs, nuts, and herbs, add a splash of cider or brandy, and slow-roast them in the oven at 325 degrees for about an hour or until the onion is tender and no longer fresh-crisp. Or take onion halves, run a skewer through them sideways to hold the sections in place, brush with olive oil, sprinkle with plenty of salt and pepper, then place them off to the side (or on low heat) on the barbecue, and grill, turning occasionally, about an hour or until softened; this is particularly good with Walla Walla sweet onions. Mmmm ...

. . . .

Onion Syrup

In the kitchen apothecary, onion syrup makes a good expectorant and old-time remedy for sore throats, and it is very easy to prepare. Take a large yellow or white onion, chop well, and place in a jar large enough for the onion plus a good inch or two of headspace. Cover it with honey, and stir well. Put a lid on the jar or simply cover with a small tea towel, and set it aside on the counter. Let this mixture steep for a couple hours until the onion starts giving off its juices into the honey, stirring occasionally. Once the syrup is quite liquidy, you can strain it into a bottle for dispensing. Adults can take one or two teaspoons as necessary, children one-half to one spoonful, according to body weight; do not give this honey syrup to babies under one year old. Don't make more than you can use in a couple days.

As for the leftover onions, how about slicing up two or three peeled and cored cooking apples, sautéing them in a little butter over medium heat for five minutes, then adding the onions; reduce heat to low, cover for twenty minutes or until tender, and serve. Try not to let the onions go to waste!

All In Good Company

I probably don't have to tell you all the delicious ways you can eat alliums—the lovely potato and leek soup with bacon, the delightful mushroom quesadillas scattered with chive blossoms, the thick slice of red onion on a fresh-grilled buffalo burger ... I want you to know that eating alliums can make you healthy, wealthy, and wise. Healthy because they're good for you in many ways, wealthy because good food is worth more than money, and wise because my mom always told me that onions make you smart—which, if you hang out with the allium bunch, you will be.

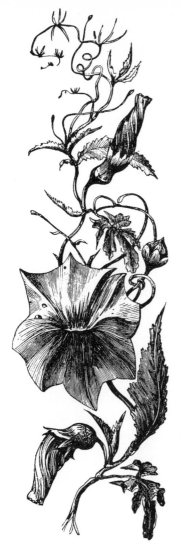

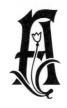

is for Anise —
no, it's not licorice

And it's not star anise (*Illicium verum*) either, which actually looks like a woody, dark brown star, is a member of the magnolia family, and is often used in Asian cooking. No, the anise we're discussing here is an ancient spice that has been cultivated for thousands of years by the Egyptians and Greeks, and the Romans used it in wedding cakes as a symbol of continuing love. Often referred to as aniseed, its flavor is similar to licorice, but the two plants are not even remotely related. Anise is part of the Umbelliferae family, which includes parsley and carrots; licorice is a member of the Leguminosae family, or the pea and bean family. I am amazed at the similarity of flavors (including that of star anise), and yet, anise has a flavor all its own. While the feathery leaves are edible, the seed is the part most often used in cooking and home remedies.

49

This tiny seed seems to be just the thing for mama and baby. Anise has been used as a galactagogue, an herb that helps bring on mother's milk, and it has also been used as a gentle antispasmodic and carminative, useful for relieving gas and baby's colic. You can simply chew on a few of the seeds to aid digestion, which gives sweet breath in the process. One of my favorite remedies is hot milk and honey with crushed aniseed as a sleepytime toddy, which I've read is an old Dutch remedy. Heat 1 pint milk with 2 teaspoons crushed aniseed until piping hot (do not boil), then strain into a large mug with a scant teaspoon of honey. Anise has been used to make cough-suppressant lozenges.

The leafy fronds are said to protect you from bad dreams if you tuck them into a soft pillow. See page 294, "X is for Xanadu," to learn more about dream pillows.

Anise is an ingredient in several popular liqueurs, including Ouzo, Pernod, Chartreuse, and of course Anisette, as well as an unusual anise and rosehip combination. It is also one of thirty ingredients in a centuries-old concoction called Trenterbe, which, with herbs ranging from anise, bay leaf, and coriander seed to rhubarb stalk, orris root, and Fuller's teasel, has "a distinctive taste and bouquet as well as excellent digestive qualities." You can find this and many other unusual and intriguing recipes, some of which include anise, in *Liqueurs for All Seasons* by Emilio Cocconi, which was originally published in Italy in 1974. All these tasty sipping treats may be why some call anise an aphrodisiac. Anise is also said to attract dogs the way catnip does cats, which can't say much for the aphrodisiac effect since dogs sniff out things we really don't want to discuss in mixed company.

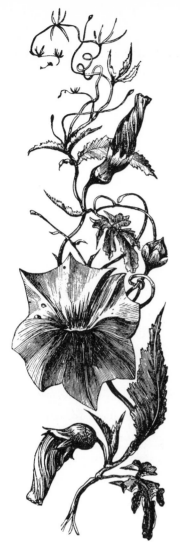

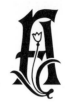

is for Apple

The apple is an ever-present staple item in our produce basket. They offer variety in flavor, texture, and aroma. Apples can also be tasty and soothing medicine if our bodies get tired out or injured. They can help flush the system clean and may even inhibit the growth of certain microorganisms.

Researchers from the Bureau of Microbial Hazards in Ottawa discovered that fresh apple juice showed strong antiviral activity on viruses such as polio. These components are found in the pulp and skin; apple cider and wine showed a lesser degree of activity, while long storage of the juice and exposure to heat greatly reduced this activity. Fresh grapes and fresh grape juice also show antiviral activity.

Archaeologists have found the remains of apples in Stone Age villages in Switzerland and Austria. The apple was cultivated along the Nile River as early as 1200 BCE. A temperate fruit originating in

Eurasia, over two thousand known and cultivated varieties of apples descend from the wild crab apple. The first apple trees in North America arrived in the early seventeenth century. If you've ever noticed the resemblance in form or flavor between rosehips and apples, it's because apples are a member of the Rose family.

Eating raw apples stimulates the gums, and eating an apple at bedtime is said to give sweet breath in the morning. Apples stimulate the liver, colon, spleen, and kidneys; the pectin helps aid digestion. Soft apples can be eaten for a laxative effect—as anyone with black bears in their orchard will attest to—while a one- or two-day fast (exclusive diet) of less-than-ripe apples will remedy diarrhea. Apples are the perfect snack for kids of all ages, as the natural fruit sugar passes into the bloodstream for quick energy without a sugar rush.

Apple pulp can be used as a poultice on inflammations and swellings such as nettle's rash, hives, or insect bites and stings. To make an apple pulp, simply grate enough freshly washed apple against a box grater until you have enough to cover the site, about one tablespoon for a sting, and place this pulp directly on the site for about fifteen minutes; this is a simple poultice. As an even quicker remedy on the hiking trail, just take a bite of apple, chew it up a little, and plaster this to the sting or scrape or whatever. Large areas such as for sunburn would be better remedied by using a so-called plaster: spread the grated apple pulp (in this case one or two cups) between two layers of gauze or cheesecloth (cut to size for the area to be treated), and carefully lay this cloth over the shoulders or back or wherever the sunburn is located; leave on for about fifteen minutes or until it starts to feel better.

When diluted with water by half, apple cider vinegar is a good wash for sunburn (of course, an ounce of prevention...). To soothe and soften the skin, you can apply this half-and-half dilution with a washcloth to the face and neck, or lay across the forehead to reduce fatigue. Undiluted apple cider vinegar also makes a good compress for gout; just pour some onto a soft cloth and wrap around the affected area, rewetting it every ten minutes or so until the pain subsides. See the section "V is for Vinegar" on page 277 for more ways to use apple cider vinegar for food as well as home remedies.

One way to enjoy apples along with other seasonal harvests is to make this revved-up relish to serve with roast pork or spicy lamb curry. I have experimented with different scented mints for this recipe, including apple mint (which I didn't care for in this dish) and peppermint (which was too strong), and found that a stem or two of pineapple mint is a good addition to the spearmint, which to me tastes best here, sweet and refreshing. Check out "M is for Mint" on page 208 for more about this fragrant family.

. . . .

Apple Mint Relish

> 2 cups spearmint leaves (do not use the
>   coarse stems), chopped fine
>
> 1 large tart apple, cored, peeled, and chopped fine
>
> ½ cup finely chopped sweet onion
>
> 1 or 2 jalapeño peppers, seeded and minced
>
> ¼ cup lemon juice
>
> ¼ cup olive oil
>
> Pinch of sugar
>
> Salt and pepper

Combine mint, apple, onion, and jalapeños in a bowl. In a separate bowl, mix the lemon juice, olive oil, sugar, and seasonings, then pour over apple mixture and toss. Serve at room temperature.

Apple blossoms have been used to make a fragrant wine, and an infusion (medicinal tea) of the blossoms has been used for sore throats and colds. I suggest taking the blossoms from a very overgrown tree; otherwise, you will end up picking off potential fruit. I have found several online sites with recipes for floral wines, and Steven A. Krause has explored this and other interesting concoctions in *Wine from the Wilds*.

In *The Herb Book*, John Lust says that the dried peels of apples were used as a tea for "rheumatic illness." Mrs. M. Grieve, in *A Modern Herbal*, says that a mild apple beverage is drunk cool for feverish conditions.

· ·

Apple Water

Take 3 to 4 whole unpeeled apples, slice thin, place in a large saucepan with 2 quarts of water, and bring to a boil; reduce heat, then simmer until soft, about 20 minutes. Strain, stir in 2 tablespoons honey, then cool to serve. Drink throughout the day as needed. This brew keeps for 2 days refrigerated, but you will likely drink all of it the first day.

Apple cider was an important staple in the colonial American kitchen. Families and villages would keep barrels upon barrels of it during the cooler fall and winter months of the year. Good cider is made from a combination of several apple types; hard cider has been fermented from this luscious nectar. From there, the savvy colonial housewife would make apple cider vinegar. Most of the apples grown in America today are created by grafting scion (a branch cutting) onto specific rootstock; rarely are apples started from seed on purpose. An apple called a pippin, however, such as Cox's Orange Pippin, most likely originates from a seed, or pip. If it hadn't been for the visionary John Chapman—fondly remembered by the name of Johnny Appleseed—the hundreds of orchards in Pennsylvania and Ohio would have matured decades later (it takes about twenty years for a standard apple tree to reach full maturity; the young trees we buy at a nursery are already four to seven years old!). Chapman procured his seed from the village cider press, which was not uncommon for the day. Around 1800, he literally led the way across the so-called Western frontier, clearing brush, planting apple seeds, then getting someone to tend the infant orchard in his stead. Then on he'd go, in his simple garb and long hair, an itinerant wanderer with humble personal needs. His obsession with starting apple trees from seed is not only legend: he is considered the patron saint of orchards.

The curious custom of Wassail—from the Anglo-Saxon *wes hal*, meaning "be whole" or to drink "to the health" of—is a midwinter toast to the apple orchard, and possibly dates back to the fifth century; some believe it is a relic held over from Roman sacrifices to Pomona, goddess of fruit. It was certainly practiced in the West Country of England up until very recently, and many neopagans and period-revivalists still do so—and why not? The tradition took place on Twelfth Night, usually around January 5. A biscuit or cake doused with cider was laid on a tree branch, doused again, and then all the folks who had gathered in the orchard would sing carols or hymns—"Hats full! Caps full! Bushel-bushel-sacks full!"—and bang pots and pans together, with the men sometimes shooting their guns into the air, generally making a great noise to ward off uninvited bad spirits and to let the beneficent spirits know where the apple trees were. The wassail bowl was sometimes passed around and shared as a "loving cup" or was brought door to door to wassail the neighbors and their homes. Sometimes even beehives were wassailed. Proclaiming a toast to those things in life that are vital and necessary, such as food and friends, makes a lot of sense, and we can see that wassail is an activity as well as a food item. Some recipes for wassail feature baked apples floating around the punch bowl. Most wassail recipes include brandy, stout, or some kind of alcohol, although you could certainly make it without. There are several recipes to be found online.

An apple decoratively studded with cloves was the original pomander, which makes sense since the apple is a pome-type fruit. In his book *Magical Aromatherapy*, Scott Cunningham reminds us that "any and all 'apple blossom essential oils' you may see in stores are synthetic [because] no true essential oil is available." He suggests that come spring you find yourself an actual apple tree in bloom and inhale the fragrance, "breathing in peace, contentment, and freedom from worry." Visualize all negative thoughts coalescing as you breathe in the fragrance, and as you exhale, dispel them to the four winds to be transformed (just do it—your neighbors already wonder about you anyway).

Indeed, the very sight of apple blossoms gives one a feeling of exuberance and joy, and a tree of ripened apples gives us pause to appreciate the turning of the seasons, realizing that "the love we share has ripened like an orchard full of apples," or so goes a not-so-old song. It's no wonder that apples were once hung on the Yule tree for winter solstice celebrations, a symbol not only of the continuity of life, death, and rebirth but also of the awesome fertile planet Earth, our mother home. It would do us well to contemplate the apple more often.

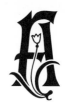

is for Aromatherapy —
makes scents to me!

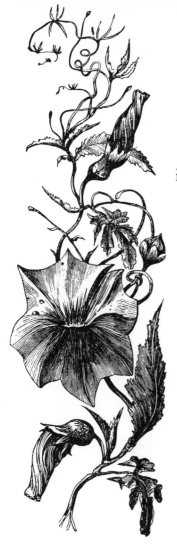

The smell of a thing is rarely forgotten. The aroma of cinnamon and molasses may transport you to your grandmother's kitchen (for me it's Parmesan cheese and parsley); the cedar chest where she kept her linens; the sandalwood incense she burned in the Buddha dish; sitting in her lap and breathing her sweet smell …

The inspirational speaker and writer Helen Keller, robbed of vision and hearing as a child, became so aroma-sensitive that she could guess the occupation of passers-by. Olfactory experiences may be fleeting and mystical like a daydream, but their effect is sustained and unforgettable. Some researchers believe this phenomenon is caused by odor "imprinting," wherein certain aromas remind us of people, places, or things. Each person is born with their own personal smell-print, and odors seem to affect our memory and perhaps even our learning processes. The sense of smell is of such evolutionary significance that the cerebral hemispheres of the brain were once mere buds on the olfactory stalks.

Our Sense of Smell and How It Works

Strategically located over the mouth, where it can survey all substances that enter, the nose reacts to gaseous molecules carried on the air. We need only eight molecules of an airborne substance to trigger an impulse in one of the exposed nerve endings, but forty nerve endings must be stimulated before we actually smell anything. Unlike other neurons (nerve cells) in the body, many of which are injured or destroyed over time, these cells are replaced every thirty days or so.

Our sense of smell is ten thousand times more sensitive than our sense of taste, and about 80 percent of what we "taste," we really smell. We can actually taste only four flavors — sweet, sour, salty, and bitter; some researchers add alkaline and metallic to the list, and the foodies among us add pungent and golden. Everything else we call a flavor is really an odor. The average sheepdog can smell forty times better (and more) than we can!

The effect of smell is immediate and potent. Smells trigger powerful images and emotions before we even have time to consider them. The smell of a person, place, or thing triggers an electrical signal, which moves directly to an ancient part of the brain called the rhinencephalon, literally the "nose-brain." The rhinencephalon is part of the limbic system, where all basic life processes are regulated, such as heartbeat, respiration, body temperature, and blood-sugar levels; it is the brain center where memories are activated and is part of a primitive network of nerves that govern the fight-or-flight response, as in "the smell of danger," as well as sexual impulses. In some places — Borneo, Burma, and India, for example — the word for *kiss* means "smell." A kiss can certainly be thought of as kind of prolonged smelling, and it has been observed that frequent prolonged smelling seems to make men's beards grow faster.

If your partner ever comes back from four days of elk camp, all tired and dragged out, and mistakenly says "it's good to smell you" instead of "see" you, well, maybe he really meant it! The so-called chemistry between lovers could be considered a response to acceptable phero-mones, or specialized aromatic chemicals secreted by one individual that affects the sexual physiology of another. It's a well-known phe-nomenon that a male moth will fly for miles on the wind of a single ripe female in order to mate. An experiment was once conducted in a waiting room where a chair was doused with male sex hormones. Men tended to avoid the chair, while women took the seat much more often.

Scent Classification

Most classification systems seek to relate the effect of scent on emo-tions, while others classify scents by the similarities of their aromas. The response to scent is so subjective, it is difficult to duplicate any anticipated results in a lab. One system developed by a perfumer sev-eral years ago is based on emotional responses. Naturally, many plants fall into more than one category.

SEX-STIMULATING aromas are usually wax- or fat-based, which when undiluted can be fairly unpleasant but when diluted "bloom" into low, sweet, deep, or warm fragrances suggestive of body heat. Musk, ambergris, and civet are examples; unfortunately for the animals, very few plants carry this effect, but synthetics are available that often come close.

INTOXICATING fragrances, such as jasmine and ylang ylang, are usu-ally floral, sweet, heady, and soft. They create languor and relaxation, dulling the senses and slowing reactions. In excess, they can cause headache or nausea.

REFRESHING aromas have a sharp, clean, high, and piercing quality, such as mint, lavender, evergreen, citrus, and camphor. These scents stimulate and awaken, and large amounts can clear the sinuses. Rose-mary and eucalyptus are other examples.

STIMULATING aromas are similar to refreshing but tend to be more bitter, dry, or spicy in quality; woods, mosses, seeds, roots, resins, and some leaves fall into this category. They are said to invoke intellectual and physical stimulation. Mint and eucalyptus are included in this category (as mentioned, some plants fall into more than one category), as are bergamot and other citrus fruits, and the fruit of black peppercorns.

Another classification system is based on fragrance quality or effect on emotions and physical sensations, and takes an either/or approach. For example, is a fragrance faint or intense, fresh or stale, sharp or dull, robust or feeble, pungent or bland?

While most aromas are subjectively described, there are some that most agree fall into certain categories, such as wintergreen: most folks will agree that it is "cool," but it is also "bright," "intense," and "animated." And when it comes to the smell of patchouli, opinions also are intense and animated—people either love it or hate it. I think a little goes a long way.

Perfume and Other Aromatics

The ancient art of perfumery has been practiced in one form or another for perhaps 25,000 years. The word *perfume* comes from the Latin words *per fumum*, meaning by or through smoke, and perfume initially referred to incense. Quite often, scented products were reserved for religious rituals. By offering pleasant odors to the gods—by burning incense—the use of aroma to induce altered states of consciousness became incorporated into rituals and religious ceremonies the world over. By inhaling the burning fumes of sacred plants, incense is thought to inspire one's mind to devotion. The ancient Hebrews burned incense in honor of Astarte, Queen of Heaven. Myrrh was burned at the Greek festival honoring the handsome youth Adonis, said to have been born of a myrrh tree. According to Mrs. M. Grieve in *A Modern Herbal*, the ancient Greeks wrote of anointing all the parts of the body with different scents, such as mint on the arms, cinnamon, rose, or palm oil on the jaws and chest, and almond oil on the hands and feet. Indeed, the first gifts to the infant Jesus were incense, and he was later anointed Christos with precious scented oils, some say by Mary Magdalene. Also known as olibanum, frankincense has historically been burned to drive out negativity and is still used in some rites of the Catholic Church. Myrrh, once used as a preservative in wine, also purifies the environment.

The most renowned perfumers in history were the Egyptians, whose complicated and mysterious incense known as Kyphi is said to be intoxicating, bringing on religious ecstasy. The Egyptian goddess-queen Cleopatra, a serious perfume devotee, was said to have met her lover Marc Antony on a barge made of fragrant cedar and perfumed sails, her palace floors spread knee-deep with rose petals. Many ancient temples and palaces were built of fragrant cedarwood, partly because it is a natural insect repellent. Islamic mosques had rose water and musk incorporated into the building mortar. Another aromatic wood used for buildings and for making ritual accoutrements is sandalwood, or santal, of which there is a red and a yellow or white variety; each are said to possess very high spiritual vibrations.

Healthful Aromas

In the ancient traditions of Greece, Rome, India, and the Far East, medications and perfumes were one and the same; both were thought to have medicinal properties. Even today, breathing the forest air deep into your lungs is still good medicine, at least energetically.

Many aromatic plants can be burned for therapeutic benefits. Juniper gives off disinfectant fumes said to destroy airborne fungi; it was once burned in hospital rooms and is most often used during winter. Spruce is another evergreen burned for clearing the air of airborne illness, and so is pine, while cedar is noted for helping clear head colds. Smoke from mullein is especially healing to the lungs; it is a disinfectant and has a long history of pulmonary use. Rosemary, one of the oldest incenses, is a powerful cleansing and purifying smoke, both physically and psychically. Birch twigs, leaves, or bark can also be burned in the same manner. If you are sensitive to smoke, all these plants can be made into a strong "tea" and simply simmered in an open pan or slow cooker (the mini versions are great for this), or run the strained tea through a vaporizer to release the healthful qualities.

I find it very practical to keep a bottle of lavender essential oil around. The aroma is both relaxing and refreshing, and I often add a few drops (not droppers) to the wash and rinse cycle of my washing machine for fresh-smelling laundry; it really does smell clean (and I use unscented laundry soap). Spruce essential oil is nice to use when mopping floors; just add a few drops to a bucket of warm water (or directly on the sponge) and mop away. I like it better than pine, although a small piece of pitch from either tree smells great when melted on the wood-burning stove.

Into the Mystic

Several different herbs are burned for their healing influence, and this means psychic as well as physical. Some of these herbs include cinnamon, hops, lavender, sage, thyme, and most resins and evergreen trees. Some herbs are combined to burn at a certain phase of the moon or time of year. Traditionally, wormwood has been burned on the summer solstice, as has St. John's wort. Rosemary is sometimes burned to bless a new home or for cleansing the atmosphere after a great turmoil. Broom flowers have been burned to calm the wind. Laurel leaves are burned to enhance divination, as in the Greek oracle at Delphi.

When creating fragrance blends, you are actually creating moods. When crafting fragrances for ritual or ceremony, these herbs and resins are blended for their vibrational qualities as much as for their aromas. As a focal point during meditation, we can burn incense or natural-scented candles to enhance the atmosphere. Many of us are familiar with Native American smudge sticks crafted from wild sage, which are burned to purify the human aura, the room or immediate surroundings, and to send prayers. It is not difficult to see that incense has been burned throughout the ages and for many purposes. As mentioned above, if you are sensitive to smoke, you can make a very acceptable and fragrant herbal vapor and accomplish the same thing. Besides, the most important thing in the spirit world is intention, and all the books and guides about magical herbalism or aromatherapy in the world don't mean squat if the scent or smoke from a sacred herb makes you want to hurl!

The following incense recipe is very easy and similar to one found in *A Book of Pot-pourri* by Gail Duff. Please don't let the kids get ahold of the potassium nitrate (also known as saltpeter).

. . . .

Lavender-Stem Incense

Remove flowers from dried lavender stems and save for another use. Soak the stems in a water/potassium nitrate bath, 1 cup water to 1 tablespoon potassium nitrate, for 30 minutes. Remove from solution and dry completely on paper towels. Place the end of a stick in an incense holder or a jar of dry sand and light. They will burn slowly like incense. Do not leave unattended.

Take all necessary precautions with any burning object, whether they are candles, herbs, or incense, and be sure to place them on flame-proof dishes, perhaps in a bit of sand.

The following books are a good place to start if you'd like to read more about aromatherapy, natural scents, magical herbalism, and our never-ceasing-to-amaze human physiology:

- *A Natural History of the Senses* by Diane Ackerman
- *Cunningham's Encyclopedia of Magical Herbs* and *The Complete Book of Incense, Oils & Brews* by Scott Cunningham
- *Healthy Pleasures* by Robert Ornstein & David Sobel

- *Herbs & Things* by Jeanne Rose
- *Human Anatomy and Physiology* by John W. Hole, Jr. (my old college text)
- *In the Shadow of the Shaman* by Amber Wolfe
- *Potpourri: The Art of Fragrance Crafting* by Louise Gruenberg
- *The Art of Aromatherapy* by Robert Tisserand
- *The Encyclopedia of Herbs & Herbalism*, Malcolm Stuart, ed.

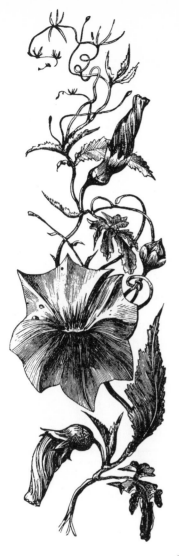

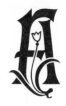 is for Aunt Cárol's
Manicotti

Aunt Carol is my mom's sister, and she learned this recipe from her mother-in-law, Lucille. Gramma Lucy was almost always at one of the many multifamily gatherings that took place when I was a kid, and it seemed as though anyone else's gramma was your gramma too. I remember her coming to our house and taking care of my great-gramma for a spell (my mom's mom's mom), and that was the first time I ever saw anyone mash potatoes by hand; I've done it that way ever since. Maybe this dish should be called Grammacotti.

. . . .

Basic Crepes

4 eggs, lightly beaten

1 cup water

½ teaspoon oil (not olive oil)

1 cup flour

Pinch salt

Whip eggs, water, and oil together until a bit foamy. Stir flour and salt together, then stir into the eggs, a bit at a time, until very smooth. Add a pinch of flour if too watery, a tiny amount of water if too thick, or leave as is (trial and error, my friends). Use either a lightly oiled, medium-sized cast-iron skillet (my preference) or a nonstick skillet, and heat to medium high—a drop of water in the pan will sizzle when it's hot enough. Using a small ladle such as for gravy, dip up some of the batter (approximately 3 to 4 tablespoons, depending on the size of your skillet), pour into the skillet, and immediately swirl the skillet around so the batter completely covers the bottom. No need to turn the crepe over; just make sure it is dry to the touch on top. Remove from pan and stack on a plate. Continue to dip and swirl, dip and swirl, until all batter is used. You can fill these crepes with the filling recipe that follows or save until next day and fill, which is really convenient. To store, simply stack, wrap in plastic wrap, and refrigerate. Crepes also freeze well.

Makes 25 to 30 crepes.

. . . .

Ricotta Filling for Manicotti

1 egg

1½ pounds ricotta cheese

Salt and pepper

1 tablespoon chopped fresh parsley

½ cup freshly grated Parmesan cheese

Beat the egg in a bowl, add remaining ingredients, and mix well. Fill crepes down the middle using about 2 tablespoons filling, then rolling one side over the other to close. Arrange seam-side down in a lightly oiled glass baking pan, and artfully spoon your favorite pasta sauce over each manicotti. Aunt Carol says, "Don't smother in sauce." Cover the pan with foil and bake in a preheated 350-degree oven for 45 minutes to 1 hour, until bubbly hot. Let set a few minutes before serving.

In case you were wondering, the name *manicotti* is derived from the protective, tubelike, white cloth "sleeves" slipped over the sleeves of a nun's habit to keep them clean while working in the kitchen. While you can buy the large, dried tubular pasta called manicotti and stuff them, Lidia Matticchio Bastianich—reigning Queen of Italian cooking in America and author of *Lidia's Italian-American Kitchen*—prefers the lighter *crespelle*, or crepe, version. She says that "it is normal for the first few crepes of the batch to come out less than perfect," so have no fear—you too can make crepes!

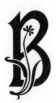

is for Barley Water

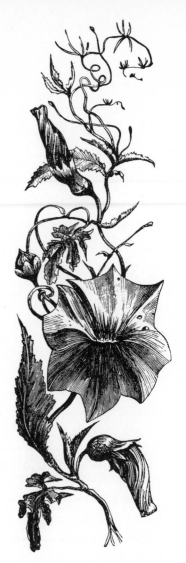

This recipe is not to be confused with barley pops or brew doggies or any other fond reference to beer. This is a remedy to be used when the patient may not be able to hold down food or if the flu is accompanied by vomiting or diarrhea. It is very soothing to the alimentary tract, including the digestive tract, because of the mucilaginous nature of barley.

To make barley water, use a ratio of four parts water to one part barley.

. . . .

Barley Water

4 cups water

1 cup barley

Honey

Fresh lemon

Add barley to the water and bring to a boil. Lower heat and cover, gently simmering, until barley is cooked, about 45 minutes. To serve, strain, add honey and lemon to taste (if desired), and drink the liquid warm or cool.

I'd like to mention that if you are caring for a young child and they are vomiting or have diarrhea for more than a day or two, it's best to get them to a doctor to be sure they aren't sick with more than just the flu. Dehydration is very dangerous for a child, and you don't want to take any chances. However, if the kid is older and just plain sick, this drink won't hurt them in the least. Just remember, no honey to babies under a year old.

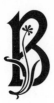

B

is for Bathing
Beautiful —
herbs in the bath

There are a lot of good reasons for taking a bath, cleanliness being just one of them. Actually, I think a shower does a better job at rinsing away the day or getting on with the day, as the case may be. Nevertheless, there are times when a leisurely, warm soak is the only way to go, and with so many ways to personalize a bath, it can become an event for all the senses. Let me show you how to make a bath a truly nurturing experience. I have limited my list of herbs to those that I can grow, are easy to gather in the wilds of my backyard, or are common grocery store items. First, I will discuss intentional sweating for health reasons, such as for fever and flu symptoms.

Fevers and the Value of Sweating

Yes, I said *value* of sweating. As you know, our skin is an organ of elimination and absorption, and sweating aids in eliminating toxins, or waste products, from the body. More importantly, when we get a fever, it is our body's way of defending against viral or bacterial invasion. As an example, the polio virus has a 95 percent growth rate when at normal human body temperature but slows to a 2 percent growth rate when subjected to temperatures between 101 and 102 degrees F. When we take fever-reducing drugs like aspirin, we impair this natural defense. Of course, fevers over 104 degrees should be promptly treated, especially in children, because high fevers could result in nerve or brain damage or inner ear problems. A classic herb combination consisting of yarrow, peppermint, and elder flowers can be made into a tea to promote perspiration; these types of herbs are called diaphoretics. The following list of diaphoretic herbs can be made into a decoction and put into the bath.

Diaphoretic Herbs for the Bath

- birch bark
- borage leaf
- catnip
- elder flower and leaf
- goldenrod
- larch needles
- lemon balm
- peppermint
- pine needles
- pipsissewa leaf and root
- sage leaf (do not use if pregnant)
- thyme
- yarrow flowering tops (do not use if pregnant)

I'd like to point out that borage, catnip, elder, and lemon balm are especially good for a child's bath. If you are pregnant, I recommend asking your midwife or obstetrician first before using any diaphoretic herbs. Make a decoction for the bath by taking one handful dried or two handfuls fresh of your herb of choice, then simmering the herb in a quart of water for about twenty minutes; strain into the tub.

I would also like to say a few words about commercial deodorants and antiperspirants. Now, I can understand why a person might want to use pit stop (how elegant), but antiperspirants, in my opinion, are unhealthy. Your body is supposed to perspire; it is one way of eliminating excess salts. Perspiration is also a means by which body temperature is regulated. To block up the ports, so to speak, is counterproductive, even if it's the armpit. (Of course, excessive sweating can also excrete important electrolytes; therefore, I recommend gentle, warm baths as opposed to lobster pots in the normal course of bathing.) Personally, I like the crystal deodorant stones; they work, they last forever, they're unscented, and you still perspire normally.

Sacred Sweating

In *The Book of the Bath*, Catherine Kanner notes, "We are born into this world after the longest, most beautiful warm bath of all." Indeed, the Lakota sweat lodge ceremony, or Inipi, takes place in a small half-dome-shaped structure that is completely dark inside and symbolically represents the womb of the Mother. The people go there to pray. Hot lava rocks are placed in a pit in the center of the lodge, and there is singing, drumming, and sweating. It is a sacred ceremony that cleanses the spirit. The Finnish sauna once included sacred ceremony as well. Steam baths and other forms of intentional sweating all have their place in cleansing from the inside out.

Bath Herbs—Actions and Effects

Several classifications, or actions, illustrate the effects of soaking in an herbal bath. Decide which herbs you want to use according to the action desired; for instance, use lavender, comfrey, and pine for a stimulating bath. To make a bath decoction, simmer one handful dried or two handfuls fresh of your chosen botanical in a quart of water, covered, for about twenty minutes, then strain into a warm bath. You could also loosely fill a muslin bag with the desired herbs, tie it shut, and take this directly into the tub. The advantage of this method is that, after soaking for a while, you can rub the herb bag all over your skin for added circulation; follow this up with a quick shower.

You might not think that herb "tea" in your bath can have any real effect, but if you consider that many pharmaceutical drugs are administered via transdermal patch, you'll realize what your skin is capable of.

What follows are several categories of herbs and their effects. You will notice that some herbs, like lavender, are in more than one category.

Stimulating

- comfrey
- lavender
- mint
- pine
- rosemary
- sage
- strawberry leaf
- thyme

Tonic

- birch
- blackberry leaf
- cider vinegar
- dandelion leaf
- elder flower
- horsetail
- nettles
- rose

Relaxation

- catnip
- chamomile
- hops
- rolled oats
- rose

Circulation (especially good for the legs)

- comfrey root
- kelp
- lavender
- nettles

All the herbs in the relaxation category, except hops, are good for children. You may wonder why I have included "stimulating" as a category after all the talk of nurturing and gentleness, peace and quiet. Well, these categories can be mutually inclusive. One can mentally relax in a warm bath while at the same time invigorate the physical body. It's not a contradiction—you may want to give it a try.

Rolled oats are a wonderful addition to any bath, providing you tie them up in a cloth bag. They are soothing to irritated skin such as from sunburn, chicken pox, and eczema. They make the skin feel smooth and silky. There are colloidal oat products you can buy and add directly to the bath, but what the heck, we all have oats in our pantry. For more ideas on healthy ways to use them, see "O is for Oats," page 222.

Another nice addition to the herbal bath blend is dried instant milk powder. Be sure to use instant (it's more of a granular product than an actual powder) or you will end up with a gloppy lump in your bath bag. Here is a combination your spirit will surely respond to favorably.

. . . .

Peace and Relaxation Soak
    4 cups dried, fragrant rose petals
    2 cups dried jasmine or honeysuckle flowers
    2 cups rolled oats
    1 cup dried instant milk powder

Combine all ingredients in a large bowl or gallon jar. To use, loosely fill a large muslin bag and tie shut so none of the herbs can escape. Place bag directly into a warm tub and enjoy.

Bathing in the Sea, Sort Of
Herbs and oats are not the only things that can be added to the bath for physical comfort. One of my favorite bath combinations takes on the fragrant essence of the sea, quite literally. First, make a combination of the following:

. . . .

Mother Salt Bath Combination
    Epsom salts (magnesium sulphate)
    Baking soda (sodium bicarbonate)
    Sea salt (sodium chloride)

Combine equal amounts of each kind of salt. Since the salts are so heavy, I keep mine in a plastic gallon-sized container for convenience. A gallon is sixteen cups.

To soak in the "sea," place several scoops (such as a coffee scoop) of combined bath salts into the warm running bath. Then take a small handful of granulated kelp (seaweed) and tie it up in a large muslin bag, and place that in the tub while it's running. Don't be tempted to completely fill the bag with the kelp—it expands to almost double, and you don't want it oozing out into the water, as it's very difficult to rinse off. Did I mention not to let any of the used, soaked botanicals go down the drain? Instead, put them into the compost. Kelp has the ability to draw out impurities through the skin while nourishing through the skin at the same time.

Not so incidentally, beneficial Epsom salts not only soften the skin, they also reduce inflammation, aches, and pains. Grandma knew what she was doing!

Oil-Scented Salts

Once you have your bath salts mixed, you can add essential oils to create your own personal bath potions. Of course, you can just use one type of oil for therapeutic effect, such as tea tree oil or ylang ylang, but it is much more fun to combine oils for the sheer pleasure of the aromas, in addition to the physical effects. Feel free to improvise, but be careful with very stimulating aromatics such as cinnamon oil, as a little goes a long way (and speaking from experience, it doesn't take a lot to make it sting!). Pregnant women should not use essential oils without first consulting with their midwife or obstetrician, and I don't recommend them for very young children either.

To make scented bath salts, you can stir everything up in a glass or stainless steel bowl with a wooden spoon, but I have found that placing the salts in a gallon-sized zipper-lock bag is an effective way to blend in the oils. Granted, you cannot reuse the bag for food, but it does work well. Put about four cups mother salt blend into the bag, then add the appropriate essential oils a few drops at a time onto the salt; reseal and shake or knead the oil to distribute. Open the bag and add more oil; again, only a few drops at a time. You are looking for a strong fragrance but not an overwhelming one; in any case, it will be diluted once you add it to the bath water. Store scented bath salts in a glass jar, cover tightly, and label.

Once you have the fragrance you're looking for, you can play with colors! No, you don't want to dye your skin blue, but a tiny pinch of powdered food coloring (available at cake-decorating suppliers) makes your creation fun and theme-oriented, depending on the fragrances you choose. For instance, if you use my favorite essential oil combination of lemon, lime, grapefruit, orange, and tangerine, then a bit of orangey color might be appropriate. Simply mix in the color after you blend in the scented oils. Don't use too much; you're not trying for opaque, just a hint, a whisper, of hue. (I even keep this citrus oil combo in a little dropper bottle and use it for mopping the floor because it's so uplifting and sunny—just add several drops to the wash bucket, no need to add soaps.)

Here is another fragrance combination with a more masculine tone; that is to say, it's not flowery floo-floo. Oh, and you have to like patchouli.

. . . .

Not-Too-Sweet Bath Salts

   4 cups Mother Salt bath combination (see recipe on page 75)
   13 drops patchouli essential oil
   7 drops sandalwood essential oil
   5 drops rosemary essential oil
   5 drops bergamot essential oil
   5 drops cedarwood essential oil

Follow instructions above for blending salts and oils. Three or four scoops into a warm bath should be about right. A patchouli- or vanilla-scented candle makes this bath a very sensual event.

Arousing All the Senses

I mentioned in the first paragraph that a bath could become an event for all the senses. So far, we have inspired our sense of touch, smell, and sight. But what about sound and taste? Do you have a portable CD player? Using our bathing in the sea example, one of the first recordings that comes to mind is *The Pachelbel Canon with Ocean Sounds* by Anastasi Mavrides, with its soothing music and mesmerizing ocean waves in the background; another recording I like is *Jonathan Livingston Seagull* by Neil Diamond. The idea behind the music is to connect the rational mind to our nonrational senses; since our ears hear everything even if we don't always register what it is we heard, it makes sense that listening to soothing sounds while bathing makes for a complete relaxation experience. Just be sure your electronic device is well out of the way of water—you know how splashy rubber duckies can get.

As for our sense of taste, a small glass of wine doesn't hurt, but the time of day may dictate whether this is appropriate or not. A soothing cup of chamomile tea or a nice caffeine-free spice blend helps set the mood (and open the pores) just as easily. The idea is to pull in elements that touch all our senses and reclaim the bath as the sensual, beautifying activity that it is. But wait! there's more!

Magical Me: Affirmations and Self-improvement

This is a way to use the bath as ceremony and to affirm whatever quality you intend to develop, sometimes called wishcraft. For example, perhaps you wish to increase your psychic abilities and want to send the message to the cosmos that you are open, literally, to the sights or sounds from the spirit realms. First, choose herbs that are traditionally connected with psychism (or herbs that speak to you personally in this way) such as bay leaf, thyme, or rose petals, or perhaps all of these. Gather your herbal components, charm them with words spoken in a positive way to affirm your intention, and make your decoction. Light a cinnamon-scented candle to energize the proceedings, and play music that "sends" you, such as *Rhythms of the Chakras* by Glen Velez or something by Gabrielle Roth. A cup of sweetened Earl Grey tea can assist in activating your mind and affirming your intentions. Run a warm bath, pour the herbal decoction into the tub, and briefly look at yourself in the mirror, saying something like, "I am open to psychic messages. I am aware of messages from the spirit realm. I am protected and surrounded by spirit helpers. The messages I receive from the spirit world are clearly seen [or heard]." In *The Complete Book of Incense, Oils & Brews*, Scott Cunningham suggests that

> as you step into the tub, feel the herb's energies mixing with your own. Visualize your magical goal. Don't make the herbs do all the work—invite their energies inside you and send them out to the universe (through your visualization) to bring your need into manifestation. Repeat the bath for as many days as you feel is necessary.

In this way, you have added your sixth sense to the equation, taking the bath from the purely physical and connecting sight, sound, smell, taste, and touch with Spirit to create a better you and make the world a better place.

All this from taking a bath! (And you just wanted to give yourself a pedicure.)

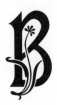

is for Blackberry—
summer's jewels

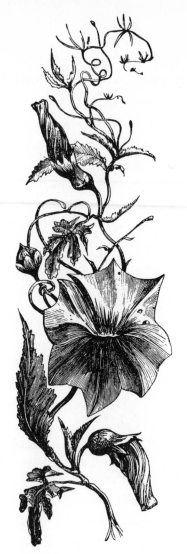

A common plant that is easily recognized, the blackberry is a trailing perennial with over one thousand varieties worldwide. Called *bramble* or *brymbyl* in Old English, and *brombeere* in German, the ancient Anglo-Saxons baked brambleberries into primitive pies to celebrate the first fruits feast of Lughnasadh at the beginning of August.

The most traditional use of blackberry as an herbal home remedy has been as an aid to intestinal rumbles. Widely used by many cultures for diarrhea because of its tonic astringent properties, a rich tea made of dried berries can be used, or you can also use the dried leaf. Take one teaspoon dried powdered blackberries (seeds and all) or one tablespoon dried blackberry leaves, add to one cup boiling water, remove from heat, cover, and steep for fifteen minutes; strain, and drink twice daily for up to two days, after which time the results should be obvious. You may wish to add a touch of honey to this tea if desired, especially the leaf.

I live where there are many types of wild berries in addition to brambles, and I also live in bear country. I have observed that eating large quantities of fresh, ripe berries, such as blackberries, will act as a laxative, for humans as well as bears.

Have you ever tried making your own fruit-flavored brandy? Always welcome around the campfire as well as on cold winter evenings spent remembering last summer's bear encounters, it makes an excellent gift if you can stand to part with it.

. . . .

Homemade Blackberry Brandy

2 fifths brandy (clean and save the bottles)

2 cups honey, more or less

2 quarts fresh blackberries (do not rinse unless very dusty)

Have a clean gallon jar ready. Pour the brandy into the jar and add the honey. If you can, put this out in the sun for the day to soften and melt the honey; otherwise, stir in the honey as best you can—it will eventually dissolve anyway. Drop in the berries, and place a piece of plastic wrap or waxed paper between the jar and lid to avoid corrosion. Label and date, then place in a cool, dry place for about four weeks, depending on strength of flavor. Shake the brandy every few days. After the suggested time, strain through a sieve and return to a clean gallon jar to settle. After two days, you can use food-grade tubing to siphon it out into storage bottles (find tubing at a wine-making or home-brew supplier), or carefully pour off, keeping the sediment at the bottom of the jar. (I strain this part again and use this cloudier brandy in cooking before I finally chuck the solids.) Decant into the original brandy bottles or other decorative bottles.

Another excellent way to use blackberries that doesn't require picking seeds out of your teeth is to make blackberry vinegar. This concoction is very easy to make and has a number of culinary uses. See "V is for Vinegar" on page 277 for how to make this and other fruited vinegars.

I like blackberries best as plain fruit picked fresh off the cane and in yogurt smoothies (freeze whole berries on waxed paper–lined trays and then transfer into freezer bags for use later). They make tasty jam (except for those pesky seeds), and they're also good mixed with apples to make fruit leather. There are several instructional books detailing the craft of drying fruits and vegetables, and your County Extension office should also have this information.

Perhaps the most delightful aspect of blackberries, in my experience, is picking them, even with (and in spite of) the mighty thorns. I remember years ago going out early in the morning with my young daughter to pick the wild trailing type called dewberries, each with our own little bucket (use plastic or enamel, the metal ones get yukky). The quiet, gentle, almost pastoral gathering of these ripened jewels was one of our most enjoyable summer activities. She would often bring me a particularly choice morsel for immediate consumption, both of us smiling, teeth stained a telltale blue, appreciating the joyful bounty so freely given by our Mother Earth.

Did I mention the seeds?

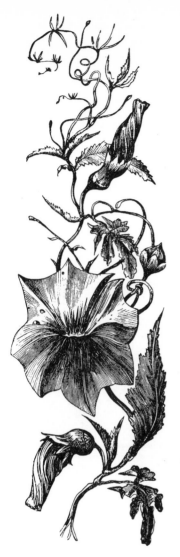

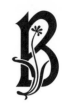

is for Brötchen —
*a roll by any other name
just isn't*

I received this recipe for German dinner rolls — the diminutive of *brot,* or "bread" — from my mom's neighbor Irene, who runs a very busy delicatessen. They serve several types of sausages, great hot German potato salad and sauerkraut, a wide world of beer, and all sorts of imported wines and other treats. I try to stop in every time I'm down visiting; I can't resist. I consider this recipe a special gift.

· ·

Brötchen

2½ cups flour, plus another ½ cup for kneading

1 teaspoon salt

1 package active dry yeast

1 teaspoon sugar

1 cup warm water

1 tablespoon oil

1 egg white

Place 2½ cups flour into a large bowl, stir in the salt, then make a well in the middle of the flour. Pour the dry yeast, sugar, and 2 tablespoons water (from the 1 cup listed above) in the well. Using your fingers, mix yeast, sugar, and water carefully within the well—do not mix with the flour at this time. Cover bowl with a cloth and set in a warm place for 15 minutes.

Add the remaining water and the oil to the well and beat dough with a wooden spoon until mixed. Turn out onto a floured counter and knead until smooth. Add dustings of the ½ cup flour as needed to keep dough from being sticky. Place dough in a lightly oiled bowl, cover with plastic wrap, then a towel, and let rise until doubled in size, usually about 1 hour. Punch down and knead for a minute or two, then divide into 12 parts (you may need a little more flour to keep the dough from sticking to the kneading surface). Shape into ovals and place 3 inches apart on two greased and floured baking sheets. Cover with a towel and let rise until double in size, about 40 minutes.

Heat the oven to 450 degrees. Place a pan or ovenproof bowl filled with water in the bottom of the oven and leave this in while the rolls bake—this is important. Beat egg white with 1 teaspoon water until frothy, then brush on the rolls. With rack in the middle of the oven, bake rolls until golden brown, 15 to 20 minutes.

Yields 12 brötchen.

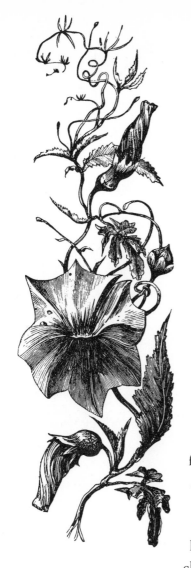

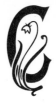

is for Camp Cook

I love to go camping; to me, it's
a lot of fun. And this takes into
consideration the fact that my home
is in various stages of completion,
is situated on a large creek, and is
already home to critters ranging
from ermine to eagles to elk to *Ursus
horribilis*. But I just love camping
out in our big canvas wall tent,
with the comfy futon and buffalo
hide for sleeping, a couple of folding
chairs, and Grandma Helen's old card
table. With a little fold-up wood stove to
complete things, one can hang out under the stars any time of year,
providing you can get to where you want to go.

The focus of any camp, of course, is the fire pit, the outdoor hearth.
Notice that the word *hearth* contains the words *heart* and *earth*, as if
the hearth, the central fire, is an earth heart. Most folks use a propane
camp stove to cook on; I have done this many times and likely will
again. However, it is my preference to cook at least one meal a day

over the open fire. It's not only deeply fulfilling, it's also fun and easy once you have the right equipment and attitude.

I once acquired a four-legged iron grate that used to be a two-burner gas stovelike thingy. I removed the antiquated fixtures and hoses and—*voilà!*—a cook stand. It has since fallen apart, so I'm scouting the yard sales for another one. I also like to use what the buckskinners call camp irons, hand-forged square iron rods, two uprights that are pounded into the ground until secure (about two feet apart in the fire pit) and one horizontal rod that rests in the U-turns at the top of the uprights. A couple of S-hooks will hold the bail handle of an enameled kettle or coffee pot. If you don't go for heavy metal, you can simply arrange some flat stones around the inside of the pit to make a level place to set your pan on. Don't forget to bring a shovel, axe, and bucket when you go camping, and pay plenty of attention to the fire and kids and so on.

Of the smaller and lighter equipment used for open-fire cooking, hot pads or oven mitts, or even leather gloves, are a must. The joys of camping are quickly forgotten if you brand yourself on the handle of the cast-iron skillet. Metal or wooden cooking utensils are best, since plastic will easily melt into something nasty. Forks, knives, and spoons go without saying; so do can openers, bowls, plates (wooden ones double as cutting boards), drinking vessels (if they're large enough, these can double as a bowl), and plenty of towels. A roll of aluminum foil can be a great help. I have been collecting enamelware from yard sales for years. A long-handled fork for sausages or kabobs is a fun extra too.

For washing, I use unscented liquid castile soap since it's biodegradable, and I normally dig a hole for the gray water, then fill it back up before I leave; I use a large enameled pan for heating wash water. The soap smell (even unscented) might attract bears, but I've never really had a problem with this. A small throw rug or thick piece of canvas is no small luxury to place on the ground where you will inevitably kneel to cook. It's as if the hearth (heart, earth) is an altar where you kneel to place offerings. With the way I cook, the spuds and onions fling their way into the libation pit with great enthusiasm.

Depending on how long I'll be camping, I try to bring a variety of ready-to-eat snacks as well as hearty food that sticks to the ribs, especially if children are involved. Fresh fruit; cooking oil and butter; salt, pepper, and garlic; ketchup; chips and lots of salsa; pancake or biscuit mix; hot cocoa mix, herbal tea bags and honey (not much of a coffee drinker); granola; jerky; eggs (hard-boiled eggs are great); yogurt and cheese; tortillas and bread; maybe even some canned chili. Then I plan my meals. What? You say I've already brought everything including the kitchen sink? Well, this is cush-camp, not a backpacking trip, and these are foods I would not want to run out of at home, let alone in the middle of—ah, bliss—nowhere. I am an expert forager and can find wild greens and such just about anywhere, but you need substantial food if it's going to be cold at night. And we don't tolerate any whiners in camp complaining they're hungry! Plus, the kids can grab-'n'-go without me having to fix them food all day (and that goes for the adult kids, too).

What kinds of meals would I, as camp cook, prepare? Depending on the time of year, usually two hot meals a day, breakfast and supper. Some folks just do the yogurt and granola thing for breakfast (quick and easy with kids), with a bigger lunch. You need to use your own judgment. My very favorite breakfast at home and at camp is scrambled egg burritos. Simply sauté a bit of onion, then scramble your eggs in. Then you can either heat the tortillas in a dry skillet or use a hot rock next to the fire. Spoon in the eggs, sprinkle on a bit of pepper jack cheese, then add plenty of salsa. Yum!

Another favorite camp cook specialty is pizza—yes, it's entirely possible. You make the dough with biscuit mix—not too moist—gently patting it into the bottom and up the sides of a large cast-iron skillet, crust thick or thin, as you prefer, remembering that it will rise. Layer your sauce, toppings, and cheeses, then cover with a lid or some foil. You need to keep an eye on the fire for this, favoring moderate coals over an out-and-out fire, and it takes about thirty minutes or so to bake. Check it every so often to see that it's not burning, adjusting the skillet so no one side is too hot, and remove from the fire for a few minutes before turning out and slicing. You can make plain ol' biscuits the same way; they are excellent with stew for supper or savory sausage gravy for breakfast. Biscuits take about twenty minutes to bake.

Kabobs are easy and terrific camp food, especially if kids are involved, as they can make their own. (Please supervise the young ones near the fire.) You can use any type of meat, cut into large chunks and marinated, as well as a colorful assortment of veggies. If you know you'll be making kabobs, prepare the meat and veggies ahead of time and store them in containers until you're ready to cook; it really helps keep your hands cleaner! If you don't have a long-handled fork, be certain to use safe, non-toxic green wood for skewers, such as maple, willow, or alder (which adds excellent flavor), and avoid conifer stems unless you like the taste of pitch. I recommend threading like ingredients with like, such as all meat chunks or sweet potatoes or mushrooms, so each can cook according to its own time. I love smokie sausages from our local butcher roasted over the fire. And yes, Virginia, you can even kabob tofu if you must.

If you can do some legal fishing where you camp, you have real gourmet fare at hand. Whole grilled trout is my personal favorite. I have also collected freshwater mussels, but let me warn you so you don't make the same mistake I did: you must soak them overnight in a bucket of cold water to which has been added a couple handfuls of cornmeal, or else they'll taste like mud. Once you do that, they'll be fine. You must also be certain the water you get them from isn't downstream from a cattle ranch and that the mussels are thoroughly cooked before consuming. Giardia (a wicked protozoan parasite) can cause terrible illness, taking weeks to overcome. Prevention is the best medicine.

Speaking of water, it's wise to bring at least five gallons of drinking water along or more if you'll be gone for a while, or two quarts per person per day as the minimum just for drinking. This is not only to avoid contracting Giardia but also to reduce the risk of dehydration in the warm days of summer. I've had heat exhaustion before, and it really hurts. Various and sundry other liquid refreshments are also welcome in moderation, with not too much sugary stuff for the kids, although those who know me well know I'm not above a Rumple Minze mouthwash on special occasions.

If it's summer, I probably don't need to tell you how to use the wild strawberries, raspberries, or huckleberries you might find, and I doubt you need a field guide to recognize them. The hucks make superb pancakes, and in a good area and year, you can easily, if not tediously, pick five gallons over a long weekend. For several years now, it has become common around here for folks to pick berries and sell them to restaurants and candy companies, staking out their claims like gold miners. Some folks are so ruthless they not only completely pick out vast stands but thrash the woods as well. Huckleberries may be big bucks for some, but for me, they are an important part of my personal food larder—and a sweet blessing given freely by the living forest. So step lightly, and remember: good food, and serving the land instead of the other way around, is worth more than money!

Meanwhile, back at the camp...

Although it's not a kitchen utensil, a guitar is the perfect entertainment for evenings around the fire. If you've been eating s'mores, be sure to wash those hands first—there's nothing worse than sticky marshmallows gumming up the fretboard! In fact, all types of musical instruments are fun played around the campfire, and even if you don't play, you can sing and clap and stomp. As you make your joyful noise and see each other's smiling faces aglow in the firelight, every now and then looking up at the twinkling stars, you realize that, even as small as you are, all time is now, and it is good. You are comfy and satisfied from the camp cook's latest marvelous creation, and you bless her, asking, "Honey, is it time for popcorn yet?"

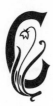

is for Catnip —
the purrfect remedy

This hardy perennial shows up in and around the garden as if by magic. The softly scalloped gray-green leaves and musky-minty aroma give testament to the adaptability of this wild, prolific, and well-known feline inebriant. Catnip is tolerant of shade, drought, and bitter cold, surviving late snowmelt, itinerant lawn mowers, and cats gone wild. I suggest that if you find it and decide to transplant it, do not put it into your garden beds unless you want a bed of just catnip; like most mints, it spreads like crazy. Like other mints, I do recommend splitting up a large specimen in the fall and planting it in several locations. That way, your cat can pick their own personal plant to chew on, roll in, and sleep under, and you can have yours. That's how it works at my house anyway.

Gently, Now

Humans can use catnip, too, if you can manage to pick off the cat hairs. First, let me say that pregnant women should not use catnip, as it is too stimulating to the uterus; in fact, catnip tea can bring on delayed menstruation. One very good (and safe) home remedy is a tea for PMS symptoms. From my own experience and observation, this is a very good tea for teenaged women because not only does it relieve the symptoms of bloating and cramps, it's also a mild sedative. Besides, what parent doesn't need a break from their daughter's raging hormones? (Probably wouldn't hurt the lads either—they have hormones too, and who isn't affected by the moon?) Crumble the dried herbs before measuring, and be sure the ginger is in tiny pieces.

· ·

Moon Cycle Tea

> **4 cups dried catnip leaves**
> **2 cups dried peppermint or spearmint leaves**
> **1 cup dried alfalfa leaves and flowers**
> **½ cup dried wild ginger root**

Mix the herbs thoroughly in a large bowl, then place in a glass jar to store and label. To make the tea, steep 1 rounded teaspoon herb blend with 1 pint boiling water for 5 minutes; strain into a cup, and sweeten with honey if desired. If you can't find wild ginger root for the recipe, substitute with dried Asian ginger root pieces or just a pinch of dried powdered ginger to a single cup of tea.

Kid's Stuff

A simple catnip tea can be used to relieve the symptoms of a cold accompanied by fever. If using for children's stomachache or diarrhea, or infant's colic, combine the catnip with fennel seed or chamomile flowers and make a very mild tea, remembering not to give honey to babies under one year old. Boil a pint of water and add a teaspoon of dried catnip and a pinch of fennel, and steep for only five minutes; strain and very lightly sweeten. A child's dose of this tea is anywhere from a few spoons at a time up to a half a cup, depending on body weight; please use common sense with this. Don't make the tea too strong or administer in large doses, as this antispasmodic herb can turn into its emetic evil twin, and it will be your fault the poor kid vomits all over everything, including you.

Even big kids can use catnip tea. I have sipped it to help relieve headaches; you can even lay a catnip compress to the forehead for this as well. Just make a strong tea and dip a soft cloth into the warm brew, wringing it out and laying it across the forehead, repeating a few times as the cloth cools. If there is eyestrain involved, lie down and relax with this compress laid across closed eyes. It's very refreshing. You can also sip the mild tea to lull yourself to sleep.

Something Sweet from the Trolley, Dear?

Catnip leaves may be candied and used as an after-dinner digestive. The procedure is simple and can be used for any number of edible herbs and flowers. It's a fun, messy project for involving children too. Any leftovers can be stored in an airtight container. First, gather several stems of catnip, remove the nicer leaves with a leaf stem attached, and gently brush clean — no need to wash. Next, have a wide, shallow dish of powdered sugar ready. Whip up an egg white with a drop or two of water until soft peaks form; give the leftover raw yolk to your cat. Using a soft, new paintbrush and holding on to the stem, completely paint each leaf with egg white, then sprinkle with or dip into the sugar, shaking off the excess. Set to dry on a wire rack, which can take a few hours. Then serve on a pretty plate after your dinner of chicken and dumplings or other rich comfort food.

Mee-yow!

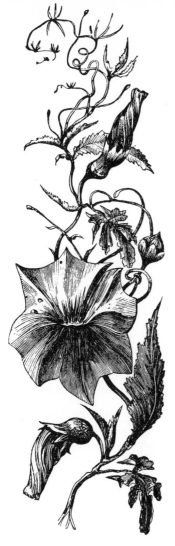

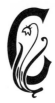 is for Cedar—
did someone say…?

Once upon a time, there was a crafty wood wizard who built a lovely chest of drawers out of cedar. His beloved wife rubbed a bit of cedarwood oil inside the drawer boxes, and to bless the project, they burned some California cedar incense to send their prayers to the spirit world.

Would you believe that each of the three times I just used the word *cedar*, I was referring to three distinct trees?

One at a Time

The cedar used for the chest of drawers was our local *Thuja plicata*, also known as Western red cedar and giant arborvitae ("tree of life"). The wood for the project came from trees on our land here in northern Idaho.

The red cedarwood oil we used was an essential oil from a large herb company who listed its source as *Juniperus virginiana*, which is also known as Eastern redcedar, Carolina cedar, Virginia cedar, pencil cedar, red juniper, and red savin. This same herb company also offered cedar leaf oil, *Thuja occidentalis*, sometimes called American arborvitae or white cedar; and yet another oil, Atlas cedar, *Cedrus atlantica*, also known as Blue Atlas cedar, which is closely related to Cedar of Lebanon, *C. libani*, and inspiration to Kahlil Gibran, beloved author of *The Prophet*.

The aromatic California incense cedar is botanically known as *Calocedrus* ("false cedar") *decurrens*. At one time, botanists gave this tree the genus name *Libocedrus*, but genetic differences were discovered in the early twentieth century among specimens found around the Pacific Rim, and so the name was changed to reflect this observation.

Be it known that no "true cedars"—genus *Cedrus*—are native to North America. True cedars are native to the eastern Mediterranean, northern Africa, and the Himalayas. True cedars have needlelike leaves, similar to a *Larix*, also known as larch or tamarack, in appearance, even though the larch is deciduous (a conifer that loses its needles). True cedar is quite dissimilar to our local *Thuja* cedar with their scalelike leaves.

Are You Kidding Me?

To make matters more confusing, the widespread Rocky Mountain juniper, *Juniperus scopulorum*, is sometimes called Rocky Mountain red cedar because of its strong resemblance to its eastern cousin *J. virginiana*. Then there are its other cousins *J. communis*, or common juniper, and the locally regional (local to me at least) *J. occidentalis*, or western juniper, which mostly hangs out with sagebrush (a whole 'nother saga) and the stately ponderosa pine. There is even a tree known as Alaska cedar, *Chamaecyparis nootkatensis*, sometimes called Nootka false cypress, yellow cedar, and Alaska yellow cedar, which restricts itself to the northern Pacific coastal areas.

Could You Please Make Up Your Mind?

Some herb crafters sell smudge bundles that often contain cedar and sage. Now, the sage could be of the genus *Artemisia*, or it could be *Salvia*, to which our common garden sage (think turkey stuffing) belongs. (See "S is for Sage," page 248, for more about this venerable herb.) However, since many smudge bundles come from the Southwest, the cedar is likely to be one of the many species of juniper, at least six of which grow in New Mexico. Because neither plants nor animals acknowledge arbitrary human boundaries (and therefore cross state lines), it is possible that the smudge bundle could actually be a juniper and sagebrush (*Artemisia*) bundle. Nevertheless, people will continue to call juniper "cedar" and arborvitae "cedar," while calling the false cedar and the false cypress both "cedar" as well.

I'm So Confused ...

Aside from burning the leaf as a healing smoke, cedar has been used in other ways as medicine (see page xxi, "Author's Note On Taking Herbal Remedies," for how I define this term). Some Native Americans used *Thuja* as a tea for headache, and the leafy branches were simply moistened, warmed, and laid to the forehead—I really like this idea. Native women were also known to use a tea of the inner bark to promote menstruation. (Please be advised that the essential oil from any type of cedar is abortive and can be extremely toxic; do not use internally under any circumstances.) As for the junipers, Native people in the Missouri River region used the leaf and berries as a decoction for colds and coughs, and sometimes inhaled the smoke from it for the same purpose. While Blackfoot Indians used juniper berries as a treatment for kidney ailments, herbalist Michael Moore says, "Juniper should not be used where there is a kidney infection or chronic kidney weakness," as the natural oils could be "uselessly irritating."

Crafting soaps, candles, potpourri, insect repellents, incense, salves, and ointments is a good way to use cedar of any type, as the aroma is quite wonderful, and it is a useful antiseptic. You can make a cedar salve by gently simmering the leaves in olive oil until rich and fragrant, then adding beeswax to thicken. See "The Kitchen Apothecary," page 3, for details on making herbal salves.

Cedar Is a Tone Wood

Alaska yellow cedar (*Chamaecyparis*) is very popular for making Native American–style hand drums. The wood is skillfully bent into a round frame, and wet rawhide is stretched across it to make a drum that you strike with a beater. The diameter and depth of the frame determine the tone of the drum, as do the thickness and type of the dried rawhide skin. Besides furniture, the wood wizard (aka my husband) also built a guitar with Western red cedar for the top of the body (the sides are big leaf maple). He found the wood out in the creek after winter washed a large stump down from the mountains, left over from a logging operation many years ago. I am so lucky that my partner the wizard is skilled in the ways of wood and can turn what looked like a washed-up hunk of rip-rap into an enduring musical instrument.

Prayers Sent on Smoke

If you like to burn incense or smudge for sacred or even practical reasons, the cedars and junipers, by whatever name you call them, might be your first choice. Use the smoke to consecrate your work and yourself with a tradition older than memory, facilitating the creation of blessed energy here and now.

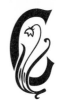

is for Chamomile—
Mother Rabbit's remedy

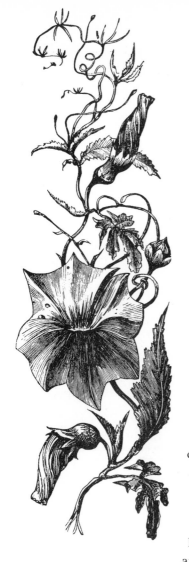

There are two types of chamomile, and both have a fragrant, applelike aroma. One is the low-growing Roman chamomile, a perennial ground cover. The other is German chamomile, a delicate, lacy annual that grows to over two feet and is a common herb for teas. Another related plant that grows in my yard, pineapple weed, is also low growing and very fragrant, although its flowers don't have circular, raylike petals.

The genus name for the annual chamomile is *Matricaria* and is related to the Latin word *mater*, meaning "mother," and *matrix*, "womb." Chamomile tea is a well-known remedy amongst grandmas and other wise women to give to their loved ones for a tummy ache, and Peter Rabbit's mama knew to give him some for his aching head. To make a mildly sedative tea for feverish children, take one teaspoon dried chamomile flowers and one teaspoon fennel seed, and steep in one pint boiling water for five minutes only—don't make chamomile tea too strong. Strain and sweeten with a little dab of honey, and have the child take tiny sips of the warm tea every now and then. Simple chamomile tea is also renowned for relieving the pain and spasm of gas or colic, relaxing the smooth muscle of the intestine. I first learned about chamomile from my Auntie Babe sending me to the pharmacy for some for my own baby's colic. Do not give honey to babies under one year old.

Chamomile is anti-inflammatory and useful for menstrual cramps. The plant is very popular in medicinal preparations, especially in Europe. Often spelled camomile and sometimes called ground apple, this herb was called *Alles zutraut* in Germany, meaning "capable of anything"—much as ginseng is considered in China. The tea makes a good hair rinse for blond hair (see page 197, "L is for Lustrous Locks," to learn about other herbs for the hair) and is also a useful bath herb. The simple tea can be preserved with a little prepared witch hazel and used as a skin toner. You can also use the plain tea to make an eye compress—or just use two steeped, cooled tea bags, one for each eye. Chamomile essential oil is said to cause the brain to release neuro-chemicals of a sedative nature.

While the flowers are edible, they may cause an allergic reaction in some. If this is not a problem for you, you might try your hand at chamomile tea jelly, something I have yet to make. The plant has been used to make aperitif liqueurs, and the "little apple," or *manzanilla* in Spanish, is also used to flavor sherry and chamomile-citrus wine.

A popular medieval strewing herb, chamomile makes a good garden companion that doesn't mind getting stepped on. It has even been called the garden's physician. You can use a mild tea to spray on vegetable seedlings to prevent damping off, a very disappointing phenomenon (see Glossary).

Chamomile is easy to grow and is a very pretty background plant. There are even double-flower cultivars. It is safe to grow around children, and they can even grow some in their own Peter Rabbit garden, along with lettuce, carrots, and peas. How sweet!

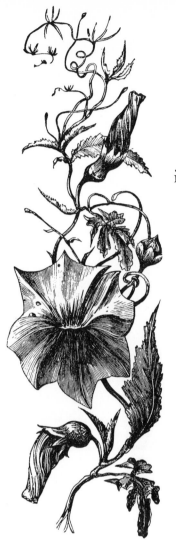

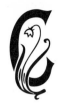

is for Chicken Soup—
for beginners

There are as many methods for making chicken soup as there are cooks in kitchens. This fact, when combined with a little forethought and necessity being the mother of invention, multiplied by the safe leftovers remaining in your fridge and the roasted chicken carcass just begging for a lemon-thyme jacuzzi, is often all it takes to dish up what trendy chefs call the ultimate comfort food.

There are a lot of good reasons to eat chicken soup, the most obvious being hunger and pure sensual pleasure. But there are nutritional benefits as well. Even though it seems watery, the nutrients from the veggies, herbs, and meat are all over the place in that kettle. If you take raw chicken bones and add a glug of your favorite herbal vinegar to the mix, the minerals will be gently coaxed into the broth and you'll have a terrific "power brew"—and the only way you'll know is that it Tastes So Good.

It's Simple

Chicken soup can take all day to prepare or it can take half an hour. It just depends on what ingredients you have, what you want the end result to be, and what your needs are at the time. If I happen to be around the house all day and am in the mood for kitchen windows steamy from simmering broth, I go to the freezer and take out a couple bags of those carefully labeled "parts"—wing tips, backs, trimmed or leftover bones and such—drop them into the pot, fill with cold water, and set it on the stove. I keep it at a low simmer (do not bring to a hard boil) and skim the foamy top when necessary. You can even include an already roasted carcass as part of the potion; this adds a wonderful dimension of flavor. If you have a wood stove to set the kettle on, all the better, but here I wax nostalgic.

There are other times when we're just plain hungry. That's when the leftover bird meat and green beans and home fries can all go splishy-splash with those sautéed onions and a dash of white wine. Cover with water, bring to just below boiling, then happily simmer away for half an hour while you fix cheesy garlic bread—easy and delicious. So, no more whining about not having time to make soup!

Quality Ingredients

The first and foremost requirement for making chicken soup is quality ingredients. You cannot take the leftovers no one would eat (with good reason), turn it into soup, and expect anyone to eat it this time either. If you're making soup from scratch, this would include fresh veggies as well; those limp carrots would better feed the compost pile than your picky kids. So, unless you over-salt, over-cook (such as cabbage into mush), or burn something, it will turn out just fine if you use good stuff. Remember, chicken soup isn't rocket science, so trust yourself.

The second requirement for making soup is a kettle or pot large enough in which to prepare it. A six-quart pot is probably big enough, but I usually use a larger one, because I make a lot and I'm messy.

Secret Ingredients

There are a few things I do when making soup (or maybe I should call it stock or broth) that are not commonly done in other kitchens. One thing is that I pick a lot of greens to dry just for winter soups — wild greens such as nettles and lamb's quarters and violet leaves, and cultivated greens such as chard and beet leaf and parsley. You haven't tasted soup until you've had chicken and rice soup with dried nasturtium flowers — unbelievable! When adding the dried greens, don't overdo it — as I have discovered with nettles, the entire broth can turn rather greenish (although it still tastes good). I mentioned earlier about adding herbal vinegar when setting the pot to simmer. You really can't taste plain vinegar, but if you use herb-infused vinegar, it will add flavor to the whole. I often add one or two dried whole chilies to the broth, and/or some sliced or powdered ginger root. I have been known to use dried berries in the broth — rosehips, wolfberries, a couple raisins — and ginseng tea. Then there are home-dried tomatoes. And be sure to remember the garlic; it's good for you and it tastes good. Don't be afraid to experiment, but do exercise light-handedness when trying out new spices, as you can always add more next time if you decide you like it.

It's All in the Wrist

When making soup from raw bones, just put them into the kettle and cover with cold water. Bring to nearly a boil, then lower the heat to a simmer; you will need to skim off any foam that comes to the top. Go ahead and add a little salt, but wait until after you skim to add any herbs or seasonings; this could take half an hour. Now would be the time to add some roughly chopped carrot, celery stalk, and onion to the basic broth, and a head of garlic if you have it — yes, I said a head, or at least a few cloves. Add a few whole peppercorns. Stir every now and then, smushing up the garlic cloves as they soften and tasting for salt or any other flavors you might be looking for. Don't kid yourself about the salt part—soup needs salt; you just don't want to add too much too soon since it cooks down (concentrates), and you really can't take it out once you've put it in. When the broth is ready three or four hours later, place a colander inside a large bowl or another kettle, and strain out the bones and stuff. The trick to lifting any fat off the broth is to let it cool, then refrigerate until cold; all the fat rises and solidifies on top. This usually means overnight, but if you do it the day before you want to use the broth, it will be ready for you. You could always get one of those handy fat-separator vessels with the spout positioned low and simply pour out the fat-free broth; I have one and it works well for smaller amounts, but it's messy and it drips and the spout clogs, and you have to be careful of the hot liquid—so, use whatever works for your situation. Now that you have the stock or broth, you can make it into soup by adding meat, veggies, and so on; use your favorites, but don't overcook veggies such as cabbage or broccoli. Freeze any extra cooled broth in convenient-sized freezer containers (or process it in a pressure canner) and you have a flavorful base for rice, beans, or even plain noodles. It makes preparing risotto easy.

If you are a beginner at cooking, I hope chicken soup is one of the first things you learn to prepare. Not only is it very easy, but the reward of your patience and imagination will become apparent after taking your first tentative sips, culminating in a warm sigh of contentment … *ahhh,* comfort food.

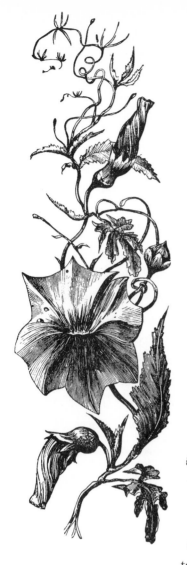

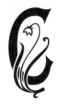

is for Corn —
*a gift from
the first Americans*

Although more and more of the country's corn crop is refined into ethanol for fuel, we can still imagine the humble beginnings of the cereal grain we call corn. Often referred to as maize, evidence shows that corn originated in Central America and the Yucatan, where it was cultivated as early as 7,000 years ago. While it took many thousands of years for it to become an important, widespread crop, Native Americans from east to west and north to south grew, stored, and ate from hundreds of varieties of corn. Most of these varieties have been lost, but thanks to the foresight of Natives and Europeans alike, many heirloom varieties have been saved, and all of these descended from the wild grass *Teosinte*.

Early Corn Agriculturists

Considering that corn has adapted to so many types of growing environments, the insight and perseverance of the early agriculturists is astounding. All types of corn—from pop, sweet, flint, dent, and flour and the incredible array of color and kernel patterns—point to generations of patient farming and intentional selection to result in such a relevant and enduring part of people's culture. Corn was planted in patches, with various types of pole beans planted amongst the stalks, while squash and melons wound their way between the patches. The squash, with its bristly stems and leaves, made a natural deer deterrent; keeping the raccoons out was another story. This trio of companion plants—corn, beans, and squash—is called the Three Sisters. All three of these plants were dried and preserved for winter as well as consumed fresh. For some tribes, "green corn" festivities lasted for two weeks, with people feasting on what we call sweet corn. People observed many sacred rites and ceremonies that were practiced during certain phases of the corn's maturity as well as specific times of the year. Among some of the Plains Indians, corn was venerated similar to (but different than) the buffalo.

Young Upstarts

It didn't take long for maize to catch on in Europe, and the farmers of New England developed many of their own varieties as well. Once they figured out that corn (a British word for any cereal grain) doesn't respond well to yeast, other types of leavening such as baking soda and eggs found their way into a wide assortment of culinary corn preparations. There is also the process of making corn hominy by treating the whole kernels with lye or ash to make a kernel that is soft yet retains its shape. Even though I am part Italian, I never tasted the dish called polenta while growing up, which I consider tantamount to child neglect; I have since discovered this simple yet sublime food, and I love it. Because it was initially cheaper than wheat and therefore food for the Italian "poor," a steady diet of corn polenta—which is basically a savory cornmeal mush that can then be chilled, sliced, and fried— led to the disease called pellagra, which is a niacin deficiency disorder causing digestive and dermatological problems as well as developmental issues. While corn does contain niacin, it is not absorbed into the body unless it is first treated with lime or ash such as for tortillas or hominy; many Native American and Mexican dishes use corn that is treated, and therefore these people did not suffer from pellagra. While we still make polenta with untreated corn, the vitamin deficiency is not so common now because our diets are much more varied.

Tastes like Home, Wherever That May Be

From fritters to spoonbread, from johnny cakes to scrapple and beyond, there are as many "traditional" methods for preparing tasty American corn dishes as there are grandmothers in rocking chairs puffing on corncob pipes (you'd be surprised). We all have our favorite baked corn *something*, a comfort food as endearing as mashed potatoes. Whether sweet or savory, Yankee stone-ground or soft Southern white, there's a mush-feast with someone's name on it.

Here is a recipe for a slightly sweet, moist, and somewhat cakey cornbread that is simple to make. It's wheat-free and accompanies a pot o' beans (page 154) quite nicely. Honey may be substituted for the maple syrup, but reduce the heat to 350 degrees, as honey burns easily.

. . . .

Wheat-Free Maple Corn Bread

2 cups yellow cornmeal, preferably stone-ground

4 teaspoons baking powder

½ cup maple syrup

1 cup milk

2 large eggs

¼ cup oil, such as sunflower

Preheat oven to 425 degrees. Generously butter a 9 by 9-inch glass baking dish. Stir the cornmeal and baking powder together in a small bowl. In a larger bowl, blend syrup, milk, eggs, and oil until smooth. Add dry ingredients to moist and stir just until mixed. Pour into prepared dish and bake about 25 minutes or until done. Cool slightly before serving.

I have recently discovered a comfort-food dish that I don't know how I ever survived without. I acquired the recipe from my friend Suzy, who got it from her granny. Similar to polenta, I have adapted it so that it doesn't have quite as much butter as in the original recipe, and I use organic yellow cornmeal in place of the hominy grits; still, there's nothing low-fat about it. Granny was a true Okie, knowing full well that you couldn't run a proper household without a good supply of elbow grease as well as bacon grease, and Suzy follows her granny's tradition in true form. This recipe feeds a crowd.

. . . .

Baked Grits

6 cups water

1½ cups yellow cornmeal

2 tablespoons butter

3 eggs, beaten

1 large can (or 2 small) diced green chilies

2 teaspoons salt

2 teaspoons seasoned salt, such as Old Bay or Spike, or to taste

2 cups grated Cheddar cheese, about 6 ounces

Tabasco sauce to taste (I use several glugs)

Preheat oven to 250 degrees. Butter a 9 by 13-inch glass baking dish. In a large saucepan, bring the water to a boil, then slowly whisk in the cornmeal, a little at a time, until well incorporated. Over medium heat, cook and stir the mush for 5 to 10 minutes or so, until cooked. Stir in the butter. Remove from heat and fold in the beaten eggs and the cheese, then add chilies and salts (do not be dismayed at the amount of salt, but don't be afraid to adjust to your taste). Mix well and pour into the prepared baking dish. Bake for about 1 hour or until puffy and golden. Let rest a few minutes before serving. This dish is very good reheated.

(Incidentally, the original recipe called for a "½ loaf" of cheese, so I just estimated what I thought was a good amount. This is the traditional method of granny-measuring anyway.)

Here's a recipe for a Mexican soup called pozole that is traditionally made with posole, a dried, parched corn that is stored for soups and stews. We use canned hominy for convenience, and it still tastes fabulous. The busy owner of my favorite Mexican take-out, Joel, gave this recipe to me. Everyone from money suits to dreadlocks stands in line for his food, literally. Joel took me in the back and had me take notes on how he makes the soup, and as you'll see, its flavor belies the simplicity of ingredients. I am excited to share this recipe with you. I believe the fresh, raw veggies are one of the secrets. I just about need to wear a bib to eat this heaven in a bowl. This recipe makes about eight 2-cup servings, with probably some left over for lunch the next day.

. . . .

Pozole Soup

> 2 whole dried pasilla peppers (find these at most large grocery stores, in cellophane bags)
>
> 4 quarts water
>
> 1 small onion, peeled and left whole
>
> 1 bay leaf
>
> 2 cans yellow hominy, rinsed and drained
>
> 2 pounds fresh pork butt, diced into half-inch cubes
>
> Salt, pepper and garlic powder, to taste
>
> 1 teaspoon dried oregano
>
> Thinly sliced cabbage, about ¼ cup per serving
>
> Minced onion, 1 teaspoon per serving
>
> Chopped cilantro, 1 generous pinch per serving
>
> Sliced radishes, a few slices per serving
>
> Lime wedges, 1 per serving

Rinse and dry the peppers, and place in a bowl large enough to cover with water. You can use hot water and soak for a short time while prepping the rest of the dish or soak overnight; either way, after soaking, remove the seeds and stems, and place peppers in a blender with enough of the water to turn into a smooth mixture. Set aside.

Next, in a large saucepan, place the 4 quarts water, the whole onion, bay leaf, and hominy, and bring to a boil. Turn down to a simmer, and leave it for about 20 minutes. Remove whole onion and add pork and the pasilla blend along with the salt, pepper, and garlic powder (Joel says that he doesn't use a lot of garlic in this soup). Simmer away for another half hour, stirring occasionally. Add the oregano. Check to see if the pork is tender, and simmer as long as necessary, perhaps another half-hour or more. Don't simmer too hard; I suppose you could always toss everything into a slow cooker for a few hours (after the initial simmering time) and not worry about it.

To serve, place cabbage, onion, and cilantro in each bowl, ladle the hot soup over all, and garnish with radishes and a squeeze of lime.

Corn for Handcrafts

Aside from a multitude of Native food preparations and a diaspora of corn dishes from Africa to Italy to Thailand, the cornhusk itself was used in many creative and utilitarian ways. Many eastern Native American tribes perfected the weaving of cornhusks into such items as baskets and moccasins. Sleeping mats and other types of flat weaving were also practiced, and, of course, there were dolls and toys. Crafting a corn dolly is easy to make and easy to teach to others. In fact, it takes longer to write it out and read it than it actually takes to make one.

. . . .
Making a Corn Dolly

Gather about 10 pieces of cornhusk (the long leaf will also work) at least 10 inches long. Save 2 pieces for the arms, which are made by rolling the 2 pieces together lengthwise to make a cigar shape, then tying off the roll at the ends near each hand; set aside. Next, take the remaining 8 pieces and lay them flat, one upon the other. Gather and tie them all together at the cut end, then divide the pile in half, folding each half back over and around the tied end, tying again around the outside of the original knot to make the head—basically tying it at the neck. Next, slip the arms between the body of the cornhusk, and tie beneath the arms to make the waist. The dolly's skirt drapes from the waist down in all her green glory. This girl dolly does not have legs, although you could make a boy dolly by splitting the husk below the waist into two legs and tying at the feet. Strips of cornhusk are traditionally used for tying, but string is a lot easier. With a bit of crafty ingenuity, one could easily figure out how to give the dolly some hair. Animal figures were also constructed.

Remember the Grandmothers

It is easy to see that corn is a staple grain that is much more than mere food; it is at the very core of a people's lifestyle, in many cases hand in hand with the buffalo. People celebrated the Corn Spirit with special ceremonies. They stored vast quantities of dried corn for the winter, along with dried beans and squash, the Three Sisters. Grandmas, both Native and European, cooked and crafted with corn and taught these skills to their daughters. From the paper-thin *piki,* made with blue corn and heated on large stone griddles, to thick hominy stews and the popular succotash, corn is still a sacred, priceless gift to the world. The next time you savor a corn muffin fresh from the oven or pluck a ripe ear fresh from the stalk and munch it down like a raccoon, don't forget to thank the grandmothers, for they will surely bless you for remembering.

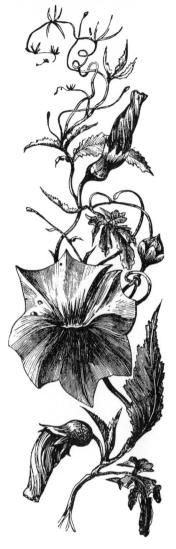

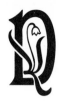

is for Dandelion—
nutritious, ubiquitous

All parts of the dandelion are edible: the sunny yellow flowers, the deeply serrated "lion's tooth" leaves, and the earthy-smelling, pale-colored roots. Even the unopened flower buds are used for food. Dandelions grow from the Arctic Circle to Tierra del Fuego. The botanical name *Taraxacum officinale* comes from the Greek *taraxos*, or "disorder," and *akos*, meaning "remedy," while *officinale* refers to any medicinal plant now or once listed in the United States Pharmacopeia or National Formulary. This very cosmopolitan, yet utterly humble weed is useful for both home remedies and home cooking.

Let It Flow

Dandelion makes one of the safest spring tonics and is one of the most common. It has been used by generations of grannies the world over. The leaf is a non-irritating liver and gallbladder tonic used to promote a healthy flow of bile, and thus digestion. Historically, it has been used to treat jaundice. Dandelion leaf is a known diuretic—the British called it "piss-a-bed" and used it to control children's bed-wetting—and is also a mild laxative, but it doesn't deplete potassium like its over-the-counter counterparts. In fact, the whole plant is rich in potassium and provides hefty amounts of beta-carotene, calcium, and iron, with notable amounts of phosphorus, protein, and vitamin C. To relieve mild edema, make a brew of roasted dandelion root "coffee" to reduce swelling of the lower extremities such as the feet and ankles. The plant is also rich in lecithin, which helps reduce cholesterol and convert fat into energy.

The nutritious dandelion root—just like its relative, the Jerusalem artichoke, or sunchoke—is easily assimilated by diabetics because of a complex carbohydrate called inulin. Both plants are in the Compositae family, flowering plants whose "petals" are actually flowers themselves. For centuries, the scholarly Arab physicians and herbalists used dandelion root to treat diabetes. I have not come across any references of whether or not dandelion is safe during pregnancy, but I would avoid using it as a tincture, which is how I usually process dandelion for the herbal medicine cabinet. Pregnant women may be able to drink the roasted root tea for edema, but please don't do this without your midwife's or doctor's approval—and a good midwife will likely know a lot more about herbs than a regular obstetrician. I mentioned dandelion tincture; I use the whole plant for making this—root, leaf, and flower—and start the process with the root first, then the leaf, and finally adding flowers when they appear; the whole process takes about a month. I use it as a general liver and gallbladder tonic. For instructions on how to make herbal tinctures, see page 3, "The Kitchen Apothecary."

The Ojibwa natives of Minnesota called dandelion *dado' cabodji' bik*, which means "milk root." Externally, the milky-white sap from the stem has been dabbed onto warts to make them fall off, but I have never followed through on this to see if it works.

It Tastes Good, Too

As mentioned above, roasted dandelion root makes a tasty brew. You don't have to "need" it to use it. The taste is similar to roasted chicory root, which is often combined with real coffee, especially in New Orleans and other places in the American South. (Chicory is also a composite flower.) Most of us are familiar with dandelion wine, some vintages more tasty than others; I tried to make some once, but what I got instead were some spectacular molds that looked more like a school science project gone awry. Dandelion has even been used to make beer, in particular a British Midlands stout. The leaves were also combined with nettles and yellow dock to make another interesting brew. I would love to experiment with making herbal beers; my husband has made many varieties of home brew, so I know I have a good instructor for when I'm ready.

Aside from drinking your tonic, you can eat it as well. In the spring, I use fresh dandelion leaves in raw green salads and in a mixed, cooked mess o' greens. There are several French and Italian cultivars available to the adventurous home gardener; just be sure to mark the ones you planted on purpose to differentiate from the "weeds"—ha ha! You can use the flower petals in baking, such as in muffins, and in sun teas—just pull them off the green stem and use only the yellow part. The unopened flower buds (still attached to the green) can be sautéed with olive oil and garlic and whatever else seems like a good idea at the time. I eat the roots that I remove from my garden beds, either chopping them into salads or simply washing them and munching them up like a carrot. Yes, they taste somewhat bitter, but they also taste somewhat sweet, just what you'd expect from a familiar wild root.

Accept It for What It Is

Many people consider dandelions to be weeds imposing on their manicured lawns like invaders on a sterile battlefield. At my home, I like to walk around barefoot, and if it doesn't have thorns, it gets to stay! I'll admit that the seed heads aren't as pretty as the flowers, and I mow more often to keep them down, but I certainly don't "round 'em up" with Monsanto or Dow, if you catch my drift. I suggest you learn to live with them (or dig them out), keeping in mind that early settlers in Canada introduced dandelion flowers to their yards to brighten things up. Farmers observed that certain plants predict the weather, and like the sunflower (yet another composite flower), dandelions are weather and light sensitive. The flowers remain fully open to the sun, but when rain approaches or the evening dew begins to settle, they close their sunny faces and tuck in for the duration.

In Greek myth, the crone goddess Hecate fed a salad of dandelion leaves to the hero Theseus. To send a message to your favorite champion, blow on the puffy seed head with a whispered plea and send the downy parachutes to the wind. Walk away and don't look back. Perhaps this so-called oracle flower will carry a message back to you … (and hope it's not your neighbor giving you the stink eye for all the dandelion seed you just blew into their yard)!

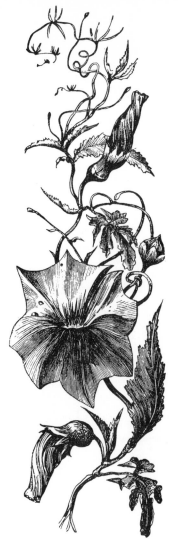

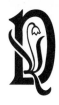 is for Deanna's Dips

No, my sister is not a dip or a drip, no no no, we just know that when she makes one of the following ever-popular dips, it's going to be yummy and everyone will love it. Our family gatherings are loud and boisterous, and the table is where we all gather to make this happen.

The first recipe here is a Mexican-inspired layered saladlike thing; second is a luscious garlic-artichoke spread; and third is a savory spinach dip (spinach—that makes it healthy)!

Mexican-Style Five-Layer Dip

In a 9 by 13-inch glass baking dish or other suitably large platter with a bit of an edge, arrange ingredients in the following order, then serve with plenty of tortilla chips. As healthy as they might sound, I think baked chips taste terrible, but do as you wish. If you're worried about fat, replace the sour cream with nonfat yogurt.

First layer (on the bottom) — 2 (15-ounce) cans
refried beans, evenly spread in the dish

Second layer — a mixture of 3 diced avocados, 2 teaspoons
lemon juice or to taste, and salt & pepper to taste

Third layer — mix together 1 cup sour cream with a half
package favorite taco seasoning; spread over avocado

Fourth layer — distribute evenly: 1 bunch scallions, sliced,
including greens; 3 small tomatoes, diced, preferably
Roma type; 1 large can ripe olives, drained and sliced

Fifth layer (on the top) — sprinkle with 8 ounces
grated Cheddar or your favorite cheese

The original recipe for the following called for half mayo and half sour cream; I've adapted it here since my husband cannot eat mayonnaise. It's nice and garlicky and completely irresistible.

. . . .

Glorious Garlic and Artichoke Dip

1 pint (16 ounces) sour cream

8 ounces cream cheese, softened

1 cup finely grated Parmesan cheese

5–6 garlic cloves (or to taste), minced

1 large (15-ounce) can artichoke hearts (plain, not
marinated), drained, trimmed, and chopped

In a large bowl, mix ingredients one at a time with a whisk, in the order given. Chill until set. To serve hot (my favorite), place mixture in ovenproof dish, covered, in a 400-degree oven for about 20 minutes; remove cover and heat until bubbly, about 5 minutes. Serve with baguette slices.

I love the following spinach dip served in a small, round loaf of bread that has been hollowed out in the center like a serving bowl. A fresh alternative to using the water chestnuts would be peeled and diced jicama, a sweet, juicy, starchy root vegetable that can be eaten raw and is often used in Latin American cooking.

. . . .

Creamy Spinach Dip
(and crunchy and savory and green!)

   1 pint (16 ounces) sour cream

   8 ounces cream cheese, softened

   1 package favorite dried veggie soup mix

   1 (6-ounce) can whole water chestnuts,
       drained, rinsed, and chopped

   3 scallions (green onions), sliced (include some green)

   1 small box frozen spinach, thawed, drained, and
       squeezed out (usually a 10- to 12-ounce box)

Combine sour cream and cream cheese until well blended. Next, blend in soup mix thoroughly. Then add the water chestnuts and scallions, folding the spinach in last. Serve with nice grainy crackers or thin baguette slices.

(Thanks, Sis, for sharing these recipes. Just remember, I'm still #1 — ha ha!)

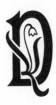

is for Dill —
*it's not just for
pickles anymore*

This common garden herb is
used for both its seed and its fragrant
leaf. Everyone is familiar with the dill
pickle, which is usually a cucumber
left whole or cut into spears, chunks,
or slices, and flavored with vinegar,
salt, dill, spices, and sometimes
garlic. And even though a pickle can
be anything from a string bean to a
peach, those long, crunchy cucumber
spears will inevitably be flavored with dill
seed. In cook's jargon, pickling is actually a process, and there is more
than one way to fix your pickle. What we commonly call pickles are
technically pickled cucumbers. You can even pickle wood, such as for
paneling or flooring, with calcium carbonate or lime.

This Fish Is Delish

If you haven't tried fresh dill weed, as the leaf is often called, you are in for a real treat. This lovely herb is used extensively in Scandinavian, Russian, and Eastern European cooking. And while the leaf may look delicate, it adds a lot of flavor. Use fresh dill weed in egg dishes, either as an edible garnish or as small amounts minced into the dish itself. It is the quintessential flavoring to a steaming bowl of new potatoes; simply sprinkle it on fresh or dollop with a generous amount of dill blended with soft butter, which you can use to season all types of fresh vegetables or even fish. Use the leafy fronds to stuff whole fish for grilling. Dill weed is an essential ingredient in a popular Swedish preparation made with fresh salmon called gravlax. The following recipe is similar to one found in *The Herbal Palate Cookbook* by Maggie Oster and Sal Gilbertie. Some recipes include thinly sliced lemon and red onion along with the herbs; I don't care for the onion, but do what you like best. Please note that Atlantic salmon is not the same as Pacific salmon, but use whichever you prefer and can procure, as long as it is very fresh. Yes, four pounds of salmon can be pretty spendy, but it makes a lot; reduce the recipe by half and it still tastes the same—delicious!

. . . .

Gravlax with Dill and Spearmint

¼ cup kosher salt

¼ cup sugar

2 ultra-fresh salmon fillets with skin, similarly sized at about 2 pounds each

1 tablespoon whole peppercorns

½ cup minced fresh dill leaves

¼ cup minced fresh spearmint leaves

Combine the salt and sugar in a bowl. Carefully remove any bones from the fish. On the flesh side, score each fillet 3 or 4 times diagonally. Sprinkle the salt–sugar blend on all sides of the fish, then place one fillet skin-side down on a large piece of plastic wrap. Sprinkle half the peppercorns on the fish, then layer on the fresh herbs. Sprinkle with the rest of the peppercorns, then match the other fillet flesh-side down onto the herbs, atop the other piece. Wrap tightly in the plastic wrap.

Next, place the wrapped salmon in a large glass baking dish and cover with another heavy, flat dish or pan, and weigh this down with a (towel-wrapped) brick or something heavy to evenly press on the fillets. Refrigerate, turning the fish package every 12 hours.

After 48 hours, open the package and drain any liquid that has accumulated. Gently scrape off the herb blend and peppercorns and discard. Carefully fillet the skin away from the flesh.

To serve, place on a cutting board and thinly slice the salmon at an angle with a long, sharp knife. Small rounds of rye or wheat bread and sliced cucumber make this dish complete, with perhaps a tiny dab of sour cream.

How Did They Know?

The word *dill* comes from the Norwegian *dilla*, meaning "to lull," and indeed, a mild tea made from the seeds is a good remedy for baby's colic and is said to help bring on mother's milk. Boil 1 pint (2 cups) water, remove from heat, stir in 1 teaspoon dill seed, then cover and steep for 5 minutes; strain and serve warm, up to 2 cups a day for mother and 2 small spoonfuls every hour for baby. You can also gently warm the seeds in milk for baby.

Chewing on dill seed is said to be a remedy for hiccups. The lulling quality of dill must be one of the reasons why it is often used in sleep pillows—you know, those little pillows stuffed with magical herbs that you tuck under your regular pillow to lull you to sleep (or, in the case of dream pillows, to inspire subtle relaxation and psychic awareness—see "X is for Xanadu," page 294). I love how folklore follows utility—or is it the other way around...?

Take It Outside

It's easy to grow dill. If you have the garden space, you can suc-
cessively plant every two weeks starting in May until the end of June
for fresh dill all summer. It is a tall plant, from two to three feet, and
prolific, so take that into consideration. Be sure to save some seed for
planting next year; before they are fully ripe, cut the stem at least a
foot below the seed head, and tie several stems into a bunch to hang
and dry in a dark, airy place. It makes a good companion plant for cole
crops–cabbage, broccoli, and so on—while growing dill with carrots,
parsnips, or other plants of the parsley family (to which dill belongs)
is discouraged. If you find that you have extra dill fronds, you can use
them in floral arrangements; they look especially nice with carnations.

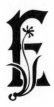

is for Eggs—
which came first?

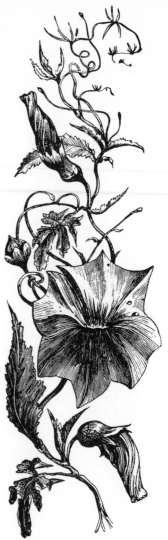

I realize that the letter C comes before E in the alphabet, but I am compelled to at least mentally place the egg before the chicken. Symbolically, the egg represents the promise of new life, fertility, creation, and even protection. Believed to have evolved from the wild fowl of India and China, it took many centuries for the chicken (and its egg) to reach Europe and Britain. Since antiquity, however, the egg has been esteemed as a magical object as well as an objet d'art by cultures the world over.

One of the most beautiful examples of sacred eggcraft is the Ukrainian decorated Easter egg, the pysanky. A painstaking process of repeated waxing and dyeing produces an intricate design of various symbols and geometric patterns. These eggs are sometimes used as amulets for fertility and protection. The word *Easter* is a form of the Teutonic goddess Eostre's name, who laid the golden egg of the sun.

These days, Easter Sunday is observed the first Sunday after the first full moon after the Spring Equinox. By this time, the daylight hours are longer than the dark, and chickens are now getting the solar-retinal stimulation they require to begin laying eggs on a more regular basis. The connection between Easter, spring, rebirth, and eggs is obvious.

As a food, eggs are a balanced source of protein (about 5.5 grams per), 68 calories, and provide a healthy supply of choline (in the yolk), which is vital to fat-based structures such as brain and nerve tissue. They also contain vitamin B_{12}. And while eggs are high in cholesterol, recent research indicates that keeping to a low-fat diet and still eating eggs shows no increase in blood cholesterol. I'm not going to jump on the bad egg/good egg bandwagon; take that up with a competent health-care practitioner. I will recommend buying your eggs from a local source, though, such as a feed store, co-op, or farmer's market; these eggs will not be cheep (oh, dear), but they will be a lot better than battery-box, mega-market eggs.

I eat eggs morning, noon, and night, though usually not in the same day. How about some quick breakfast burritos? Simply scramble some eggs in a bowl with salt and pepper and set aside. In a medium-sized (I prefer cast-iron) skillet, sauté any combination of leftover potato, veggies, or meat in a bit of oil over medium-high heat. Throw in some onions or scallions too while you're at it. Pour in the eggs and cook, stirring, until done to your liking. Of course, you have heated your tortilla over another burner and have it warm and waiting for the eggs, along with some shredded cheese and salsa ... *cock-a-doodle-doo!*

One of my favorite spring potluck contributions is a veggie frittata, which is sort of like a baked Italian omelet. The herbs and veggies available to us in spring reinforce the egg as a symbol of freshness and renewal. The beauty and convenience of a frittata is that it doesn't have to be served hot—room temperature is traditional. This recipe requires a lot of eggs, but it's cut up small, so it makes a lot.

. . . .

Spring Vegetable Frittata

This is sort of a freeform thing, where you can pick and choose from just about any kind of spring vegetable or herb for the filling—such as asparagus, broccoli shoots, peas, chives, parsley, wild chickweed or lamb's quarters or violet leaves, spinach, spring onions, and so on, even cooked potato. Bits of roasted red pepper are delicious. You can add cheese or a small amount of flavorful meat, but let the veggies be the star. To make a frittata in a 9 by 13-inch glass baking dish, you will need:

15 eggs

¼ cup milk or cold water

Salt and pepper

3 cups lightly sautéed or blanched vegetables

**1 small sweet onion or shallot, chopped
and sautéed just until soft**

1 small handful fresh herbs, chopped

4 ounces (about 1 cup) grated cheese, if using

**4 ounces ham, proscuitto, or sweet Italian
sausage (browned first), if using**

Butter for baking dish

Preheat oven to 350 degrees. Butter the baking dish and set aside. Crack eggs into a large bowl with the milk, salt, and pepper. Whisk or beat well—I use an olde-timey hand rotary beater. Place the prepared cooked vegetables in the buttered dish, distributing evenly, then the meat, if using, then the cheese. You might consider tucking in a small spoonful of ricotta here and there too—very yummy. Next, sprinkle on the herbs or leafy greens. Finally, carefully, pour the eggs over all.

Bake for 20 to 30 minutes or until frittata is set and the eggs are no longer runny; don't let the frittata get dry. Remove from the oven and let cool 15 minutes. If serving for potluck, cut into 2-inch squares, otherwise cut a little bigger for a main dish. The frittata can be served at room temperature.

The following recipe is adapted from one found in *Fancy Pantry* by Helen Witty. Pickled eggs suffer a poor image, lined up next to those jars of nasty ol' pickled kielbasa on the bar of a smoky tavern (I should write a ten-cent detective novel). Well, these eggs are a rather pretty pickle by comparison and would make a complementary addition to a cold sandwich or picnic lunch, with or without the beer.

Gilded Eggs

> 2 dozen small eggs, preferably a couple
> weeks old (easier to peel)
>
> Salt
>
> 3 cups white vinegar
>
> 1 cup water
>
> 1 (3-inch) cinnamon stick
>
> 4 teaspoons sugar
>
> 1 tablespoon dried onion flakes
>
> 2 teaspoons plain sea salt (not iodized)
>
> 2 teaspoons whole peppercorns
>
> 1 teaspoon whole allspice
>
> 1 teaspoon ground turmeric
>
> 2 whole, dried chili peppers

Place the eggs in a large pan and cover with cold water by one inch. Toss in a handful of salt. Gradually bring to a boil and simmer about 10 minutes, then drain and rinse under cold water to cool. To make the brine, combine vinegar, water, cinnamon, sugar, onion flakes, sea salt, peppercorns, allspice, and turmeric in another pan, and heat to simmer, covered, about 15 minutes. Keep hot.

Meanwhile, sterilize 2 wide-mouth quart canning jars and lids (boil them in water for 5 minutes or use the sanitize setting on your dishwasher), and have them ready. Carefully peel eggs, rinse, and pat dry, then place into the jars, along with 1 dried chili pepper in each. Pour boiling hot brine over the eggs, dividing spices evenly. Be sure the eggs are well covered with brine; if not, add more vinegar (do not dilute with water). Let eggs cool, uncovered, then cover the jar with plastic wrap or waxed paper, then the lids, and then store in the refrigerator for 10 days before serving, to give the flavors time to meld. The eggs will keep about 6 months refrigerated.

For this next recipe, I thank my ol' buddy Bullhead. "There's no substitute for experience," says Bully, as you will need to know how to make other smoked foods such as fish and fowl in order to make these unusual eggs. A little electric smoker will work, as will one of those dome-shaped charcoal smokers (do not confuse this with a regular barbecue grill—but you should already know that). This brine will cover up to four dozen eggs, depending on size.

. . . .

Smoked Eggs

3 to 4 dozen eggs, depending on size

2 cups brown sugar

1 cup plain sea salt

1 gallon cold water

Place the eggs in a large pot and cover with cold water by at least 1 inch. Slowly bring to a boil, then turn off the heat and cover for 5 minutes. Remove from heat and rinse with cold water until the eggs have cooled. Combine sugar, salt, and the 1 gallon of water in a large container, stirring until dissolved, to make the brine. Peel the eggs and place in brine for 24 to no longer than 36 hours in the refrigerator. Remove from brine and pat dry.

Now, get your smoker going in your usual way—I'm not going to instruct you how—low heat, plenty of smoke. Bullhead has used all varieties of wood chips for smoking, but I am partial to hickory in this application—it's almost like bacon flavor right on the eggs! Get the smoke going good and thick before placing the eggs on the rack. Smoke for a half hour to 45 minutes tops; do not oversmoke. I've never eaten one warm, but I wouldn't blame you if you tried. They are very good cold, however, sliced in half and served with other cold foods at a picnic or backyard barbecue, and definitely with a cold one.

I'd like to share an idea I learned as a student helper while working at Head Start. It's something you might want to incorporate into your own spring rites, a crafty, fun way to contain your eggs before, during, or after the hunt. This project is excellent for young children to make as there are no sharp things involved, it takes very little supervision, and success is guaranteed. Plus every child loves to watch things grow. Start the project at least two weeks before the holiday so it will be ready in time. These living Easter baskets also make a charming centerpiece for the table, alongside vases of nodding yellow daffodils and fragrant hyacinths in their beautiful array of colors. You can purchase wheat berries at a health food store or large market that sells bulk grains.

. . . .

A Living Easter Basket

Line a plastic berry basket with 2 sheets of aluminum foil or plastic wrap. Evenly distribute ¾ cup potting soil in the basket. Sprinkle 2 teaspoons whole wheat berries over the top of the soil. Water only once, ¼ cup, and cover the basket for 2 days while placing it in the sunlight. Remove cover after two days and keep in the sunlight. Rotate the basket every couple of days so the wheatgrass will grow evenly. Then you will have a grassy, nestlike basket in which to place the colored eggs. What fun!

There are a multitude of recipes that feature eggs, such as Russian vegetable pie, Greek Easter bread, French *gougères*, and Mexican *huevos rancheros*, to name just a few. Plain old scrambled eggs never hurt anyone either; sometimes you just need a midnight snack. So let us give eggs the standing ova-tion (someone stop me) they deserve. Just remember, he who wants eggs must endure the clucking of the hen, especially at midnight!

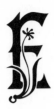

is for Elderberry—
food, physic, and folklore

The blue elderberry is a medium-sized shrublike tree often found growing on old country roads, down along fence lines, and around various other haunts of human habitation. The small, creamy white flowers grow in cloudlike clusters and smell sweet and spicy; the tiny, dark blue berries are covered with a whitish chalk on the skin and usually ripen in late August and into September. They taste sour, sweet, and slightly bitter, and have tiny edible seeds. (Do not eat or harvest the red elderberry varieties; they are toxic.) It is best not to eat the fresh fruit in any quantity, especially for children (the western species can be emetic in large amounts); they are much tastier dried or cooked anyway.

In the Kitchen

You can use dried elderberries the way you would raisins. The fresh berries can be frozen to use later in pies (freeze on a waxed-paper-lined baking sheet until hard, then put in a freezer bag or container for storage). A well-made elderberry wine is sublime. You can add the freshly cleaned and trimmed flowers to muffins or pancakes (just shake 'em real good to loosen any bugs—no need to wash). Even more delightful are elderflower fritters. Leaving the flowers on the stem for this and separating into convenient-sized clusters, simply dip a cluster into fritter batter, then into hot oil, and proceed from there. If you're lucky, you'll have some rose-petal honey on hand for a condiment (see "R is for Roses," page 240, for how to make it).

In the Kitchen Apothecary

Elder flowers are combined with yarrow and peppermint to make an excellent remedy for flu symptoms, inducing perspiration, and helping break a fever. This remedy can also be given to children, although they might not appreciate the flavor of yarrow—I don't think grown-ups like it much either (but I certainly love how it smells). You can also turn elderberries into a soothing syrup. An old-time remedy called elder rob is made from red wine mulled with dried elderberries and cinnamon and taken for the flu...very relaxing.

Externally, you can use elder flowers in the bath to calm anxiety. Wash freely with the following skin potion, also known as aqua sambuci, and use as a mild astringent for blemishes, sunburn, or any other mild irritation.

. . . .

Elder Flower Water

Fill a quart jar with cleanly picked fresh elder flowers (cut off the larger stems), pressing down to pack the jar, and then pour on boiling water to cover, leaving a tiny bit of headspace. When slightly cool, add ¼ cup (2 ounces) 100-proof vodka, cover with a cheesecloth, and set in a warm place overnight. Next day, strain and decant. Use as described above.

Legend and Lore

The elder tree is steeped in folklore. The generic Latin name, *Sambuca,* inspires the Italian word *sampogna*, a type of ancient flute. Indeed, the stem of an elder branch has pith that hollows out easily, leaving a tube to make a flute or whistle. I've heard of hunters who can imitate the sound of an elk with this stem-whistle. (Be aware that elder bark contains nauseating alkaloids if you decide to try this for yourself; bottom line, don't chew on the whistle.) Several legends tell of an Elder Mother inhabiting the tree, known in Denmark as Hylde-Moer, and that one must seek her permission before cutting down the tree. Legend also claims that if you stand under the tree on Midsummer's eve, you may see the King of the Faeries and his retinue.

Say "Thank You"

Since elder can be so plentiful where it grows, it seems like a good plant from which to reap bounty, providing you ask the blessed Hylde-Moer ahead of time and thank her for her generous gifts.

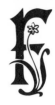

is for Fennel

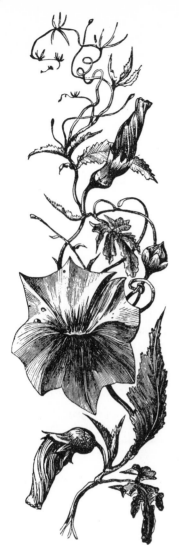

Native to the Mediterranean and eastward to India, fennel is a fragrant, warm, sweet aromatic herb that lends its distinctive flavor to many meals. Its mild remedial action is soothing and welcome.

As an herbal home remedy, fennel is most often used for indigestion and taken as a tea of the seed; the leafy herb is sometimes used too (see "S is for Spice Rack Remedies," page 255). Fennel is a carminative, which means it helps relieve gas, and it is especially good for baby's colic. Said to increase breast milk, a nursing mother can drink fennel seed tea and impart its soothing qualities to her baby in that way. Some people take crushed fennel seed warmed with milk and honey as a sleepytime toddy. The tea can also be used as a gargle for a sore throat. To make fennel tea, simmer 1 tablespoon whole, dried seed with 1 pint water for 5 minutes; cover and remove from heat, then steep for another 15 minutes. Strain and serve sweetened with a bit of honey (except if you're giving to baby—no honey to babies under one year old).

The use of fennel as a culinary companion is usually associated with steamed fish or Italian and East Indian cooking. There are two types of fennel: *Foeniculum vulgare*, known as seed fennel, and *F. dulce*, known as sweet fennel or by the Italian name *finoccio*. The delicate leaf of sweet fennel is often used to wrap or stuff whole fish destined for the grill or steamer; this method actually aids in the digestion of oily fish such as salmon. Its bulbous stalk, looking not unlike a bunch of celery, can be eaten raw, steamed, roasted, grilled, and certainly sautéed. Truth be told, it took me years to finally break down and try fresh fennel, and now I love it. Fennel seed is a complementary seasoning to lamb or pork and is an essential ingredient in sweet Italian sausage. Lentils and other beans also welcome a touch of fennel seed.

The recipe that follows is a good example of how the common potato can be transformed by the sweet, aromatic flavor of fennel seed. The venerable Idaho potato is grown extensively in the southern part of the state as well as neighboring Washington, but this dish can be enjoyed no matter where you live. I sometimes use Yukon Gold potatoes. Do not use red mashing potatoes, they fry up sticky. You will have to use your own judgment and experience on the heat level and amount of oil; I will give approximate amounts. I highly recommend using cast-iron skillets. The amount of herbs specified is light-handed; I usually use more.

· ·

Famous Potatoes with Cheddar and Two Seeds

   4 medium baking potatoes, peeled and cubed ½-inch

   1 medium onion, peeled and coarsely chopped

   1 teaspoon whole fennel seed

   ¼ teaspoon whole anise seed

   ¼ teaspoon dried oregano or tarragon (or both)

   Salt and pepper

   ½ –1 cup grated Cheddar cheese (mozzarella is good too)

Approximately 1 teaspoon plus 2 teaspoons cooking oil
¼ cup sunflower seeds, optional

In a large skillet or other heavy frying pan, over medium heat, sauté onion in about 1 teaspoon oil. After they soften, about 7 minutes or so, remove from skillet and set aside; wipe out the skillet, then add about 2 teaspoons oil. Return to medium-high heat—the oil should begin to "smile" in the skillet—then add the potatoes, turning to coat in the oil. Fry them up a few minutes to start crisping, then cover and turn heat to medium-low and cook for about 15 minutes. (It's important not to use too much oil, but to use enough; I wish I could give you an exact amount, but this is something you'll have to experience.)

In the meantime, take the fennel and anise seeds and crush them with a mortar and pestle. (You say you don't have one? Try a flat rock base with a round rock crusher. Or put the seeds in a plastic bag and crush them with a hammer on the cutting board. Or leave the seeds whole—don't get too worked up over it.) Gently crush the oregano and sprinkle the seasonings, including the seeds, salt, and pepper, over the potatoes. Cover again and cook until the potatoes are done, about 15 minutes (test a piece). Remove lid, turn up the heat a little, return the onions to the skillet, combine, and let the potatoes brown to your liking, turning once. When nice and crisp, sprinkle with the grated cheese, cover, and turn off the heat. When cheese is melted, about 5 minutes, serve to those whose appetites were stimulated by the fantastic aroma. If you toss in sunflower seeds, the recipe will be more protein-correct and suitable to serve as a meatless main dish. In any case, there will probably be no leftovers. Serves 6 as a side dish or 4 as a meal.

A nice variation that adds a tasty bit of color to this dish is to include a healthy portion of minced fresh chives or parsley or both. Chervil has an anise flavor that would also complement this dish. Add the fresh herbs at the end of the cooking time, tossing with the potatoes just before topping with cheese. Do not be tempted to purchase pre-ground fennel seed—it will be stale.

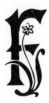

is for Flowers —
in answer to the question,
"Gramma, why are there
flowers in the salad?"

Yes, indeed, there are some flowers in the salad. Many folks are surprised to see even the common violet or nasturtium in their green, leafy salad, but people have been eating flowers for centuries. In days of olde, some flowers were pounded with sugar and eaten to dispel unseemly humours, while some flowers have been fermented into delightful alcoholic beverages — another way to improve one's *humour*. There are also some flowers that should never be consumed, which I will list at the end of this chapter. Also, never eat flowers from the florist: they're all treated with fungicides, insecticides, and other chemicals, rendering them toxic and inedible even if they're not poisonous flowers.

Kitchen Herb Flowers

Generally speaking, all the culinary herbs—such as basil, marjoram, oregano, thyme, and savory—have edible flowers. Normally, we try to harvest these herbs before they are in full flower, but some do get away from us, and these flowers are just as useful in the kitchen as the leaves; they taste more or less the same as the leaf. These flowers can be tossed into salads, minced into omelets or frittatas, and added to rice or soup toward the end of the cooking time. Thyme flowers make a good tea for chest colds and sore throats. While not often used in cooking, the flower petals of monarda, often called bergamot or bee balm, add a spicy, minty, almost oreganolike flavor to salads, and they make a snappy cup of tea, useful for coughs and lung congestion. To make a simple herb or herb-flower tea, boil 1 pint water, remove from heat, place 1 teaspoon fresh herbs or ½ teaspoon dried in the water, then cover and steep for 10 minutes; strain to serve, and sweeten with honey if desired. (Remember: no honey to babies under one year old.)

Flowers from kitchen garden herbs make an attractive edible garnish. This includes the azure-blue flowers of the borage plant, whose leaves have an aroma and taste of reminiscent of cucumber (and is put to good use in sorrel soup—see page 252). Flowering herb stems can also be used to make herbal vinegars; flowering basil immediately comes to mind, especially the purple type, as it will tint the vinegar a beautiful pinkish-purple and taste wonderful; see "V is for Vinegar," page 277, to learn how to make herbal vinegars. Another fun summer project is to take your favorite combination of edible flowering herbs—thyme and marjoram, for example—tie a few sprigs together with kitchen string, and hang them to dry for use later in soups and stews. Put these into a wide-mouthed glass jar for easy retrieval. These miniature herbal bouquets make useful gifts, and you can also string them together on a length of jute or twine to make a rustic garland to decorate your kitchen.

Sweet-Faced Flowers

As you will note in "V is for Violet" (page 286), all the violets, violas, pansies, and johnny jump-up flowers are edible, the domestic variet- ies as well as the wild. It's hard to describe the taste of a violet flow- er; it's almost anise-flavored, yet it isn't—I guess they just taste like themselves. I have used violas and johnnys in my spring salads for years; it's an annual tradition. The yellow variety that grows wild in the woods near my home blooms at about the same time as the morel mushrooms are emerging, and both are great in risotto. Sweet violet flowers make an enchanting syrup like nothing you've ever had—see "The Kitchen Apothecary," starting on page 3, for instructions on how to make herbal syrups. Many herbal chefs use this family of flowers to decorate butters and cheeses, creating something that resembles a tiny float from Pasadena's Rose Bowl Parade—almost too pretty to eat! Try it yourself sometime, or get your kids to do the decorating—they will have loads of fun. I can hear it now—"Sally, stop eating all the flowers! We're saving them to decorate the butter!"

Unusual and Fragrant

Lavender flowers don't often make it into the kitchen, except may- be to flavor lemonade (see page 188, "L is for Lemon") or in French herbal blends, but have you ever tried lavender shortbread cookies? Simply add one tablespoon fresh or dried lavender flowers to your favorite shortbread recipe, and do not overbake the cookies. Be ready for something special.

Another not-so-common flower in the kitchen is the romantic rose. There are dozens of ways to eat a rose, from the silky petals to the voluptuous hips, and if you refer to "R is for Roses," page 240, you will find several recipes to get you in the mood.

She Loves Me...

...and I love her too! I am referring to the sunny marigold, but not just any marigold. The orange-petaled flower with the golden center we call calendula is also referred to as pot marigold or, simply, marigold. Calendula was widely used in Elizabethan times as a food and potherb. The petals can be made into a tonic tea for the lymphatic system. Calendula petals are well known as an herb for sensitive skin and are often included in skin preparations for babies. A strong tea of the petals makes a golden hair rinse. You can find other suggestions for using herbs and flowers on the hair in "L is for Lustrous Locks," page 197.

You can even eat the petals of the delicate gem marigolds (of the common garden-variety marigold), and these have a citrusy aroma and flavor such as lemon and tangerine. You can take the petals of either of these marigolds and toss them into pancakes, muffins, or even birthday cakes. I have seen wedding cakes decorated with calendula petals and other flower petals (such as the common daisy), much to everyone's delight. Any of these could be folded into a tub of whipped butter. Just use the petals, as the whole flower head of any of these would not be palatable.

Dandelion petals also fall into the category of edible flower petals, and I have seen where the unopened flower bud itself was also used as food; I'm thinking a wilted spinach salad with the dandelion buds quickly sautéed in a dab of bacon grease and then tossed in—bitter, but tasty. There is a whole chapter devoted to dandelions in Euell Gibbons' *Stalking the Wild Asparagus*, a perennial favorite that is never out of style. He was known to serve dinner guests a several-course meal that featured dandelion in one form or another—including "coffee" and wine—in each course. Talk about a wild and crazy guy.

Flowers with Attitude

My favorite edible spring flower blooms atop the slender chive stem. The flavor is sweet and biting, with a crisp texture. The separate florets radiate from the central stem and are easy to snip off all at once to use in salads, soups, and scrambled eggs (one of my favorites). Nothing says early spring to me like fresh green chives and their purple blossoms; in my mind even now, I can hear the robins chirping, and I'm out there getting my slippers wet in the early morning garden, just standing there, sniffing the fresh air ... *ahhh*, life is good.

Other edible flowers that are more of a byproduct of over-mature garden vegetables are radish and arugula flowers. They are mustard-like in flavor, with a sweet sharpness and pleasant texture. I think the arugula flowers taste much better than the leaves.

Another edible flower with bite is the nasturtium. The leaves are edible also, but personally I prefer the flowers. Not only are they tasty torn up into a salad or floating blissfully on the sea of a cool summer soup, but they can also be dried and used in winter soups too. In fact, the nasturtium, which is native to Peru, contains a natural antibiotic and enhances the immune system. They also fall into the next category of edible flowers.

Stuff It!

And I mean that in a most tasteful way. Nasturtium flowers are great stuffed with a bit of garlicky cream cheese. So are hollyhocks (my Gramma Lil called them Polish roses) — just remove the large stamen in the middle before stuffing, and may I recommend a lemony-chive flavoring to the cream cheese, or perhaps a bit of curry powder. Hollyhock flower is also a gentle diuretic when made as a simple tea; it is related to the marshmallow plant, which has been used as a soothing emollient for centuries. Hollyhock makes yet another soothing tea that is good for sore throats and coughs.

Another edible flower suitable for stuffing, which must be cooked before eating, is squash blossoms, especially zucchini. Be sure to take the male flowers on the long stems and not the female flowers on the swollen stems, or you'll be robbing your plant of all the zucchini.

. . . .

Stuffed Squash Blossoms

Pick the squash blossoms mid-morning, after the dew is off and before they wilt; pick free of any insects that may be hiding inside. Do not wash these delicate flowers. Keep chilled until ready to use. Then, stuff carefully with a small amount of jack or mozzarella cheese—you'll just sort of have to lay a thin slice or two in there, and secure with a toothpick if necessary. Next, lightly dredge in seasoned flour and shake off the excess; dip into egg beaten with a touch of milk, then dredge again in seasoned breadcrumbs or cornmeal. In a large skillet over medium-high heat, fry these stuffed squash blossoms in a bit of sunflower or other plain oil, turning once, until golden brown. Serve with fresh corn on the cob and a salad for a meat-free supper, and you're in summer garden paradise.

Just Because They're Pretty...

Under no circumstances should you eat any of the following flowers, no matter if they are wild or domestic. They are noxious, poisonous, toxic, deadly, or worse. Don't even touch 'em. I'm even listing them in capital letters to show I mean business.

- ACONITE (Monkshood)
- BLEEDING HEART (and Dutchman's breeches)
- BUTTERCUP
- CLEMATIS (virgin's bower)
- DEATH CAMAS (white flower)
- DELPHINIUM

- FOXGLOVE (digitalis)
- HEMLOCK (not the tree)
- HYDRANGEA (snowball bush)
- IRIS
- LUPINE (including the seeds)
- NIGHTSHADE
- OLEANDER
- PEONY (some references list this as edible, some not; when in doubt, don't)
- PERIWINKLE
- POINSETTIA
- SWEET PEA (not the garden or vegetable pea)
- TANSY
- WISTERIA

There are others, but these are the most common. I would also advise against eating wildflowers (or any other part of the plant) that resemble the dill plant, even though many are edible, since the Umbel family—their flower heads look like umbrellas—has some virulently poisonous members in their ranks. So do certain members of the lily family, like the above-mentioned death camas, but onions and chives are lilies too, so I guess you can't judge a whole family on account of one or two members. If you are gathering wild flowers to eat, be sure to make a positive identification first before picking. If you want to eat garden flowers and aren't sure which is which, ask at your local nursery or your County Extension Master Gardeners for help in identifying the safe from the sorry. (*Oops*! Pulmonary arrest, how inconvenient ...)

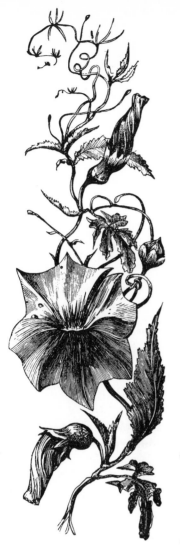

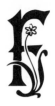

is for Fresh Fruit Pie
with Coconut-Cream
Cheese Crust

I first developed this recipe when I was in college (the mother recipe originated in a long-lost women's magazine), and it was quickly devoured by all us starving artists. In spite of all the fresh fruit (and please do use what's in season), this pie is quite rich, so now that we're fifty-something, we don't take such a huge piece. Make it for a summer brunch, a winter luau, or any friendly get-together.

. . . .

Fresh Fruit Pie with
Coconut-Cream Cheese Crust

FOR THE CRUST:

> 1 (8-ounce) package cream cheese, softened
>
> 1 tablespoon lemon juice
>
> 2 teaspoons grated lemon rind
>
> 1 cup whipping cream
>
> 2 tablespoons sugar
>
> ½ cup grated coconut (if you don't like
>   coconut, try sliced almonds)

Combine cream cheese with the lemon juice and rind, blending until smooth. In another bowl, whip the cream and sugar, then fold into the cream cheese mixture. Spread evenly in the bottom and up the sides of a 9-inch glass pie plate. Freeze until firm, about 2 hours.

FOR THE FILLING:

> 3–4 cups seasonal fresh fruit of your choice, such as
>   bananas, strawberries, peaches, blueberries (use more
>   than one kind of fruit), sliced into bite-sized pieces
>
> ½ cup raspberry jam, orange marmalade, or your
>   favorite jam (something to complement the fruit)

About 5 minutes before serving, toss the fruit with the jam. Fill the frozen shell with the fruit and serve immediately.

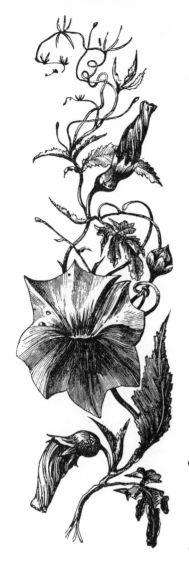

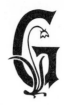

is for Gingerbread

Who doesn't love a moist, fragrant square of gingerbread topped with a bit of whipped cream or a scoop of vanilla ice cream? Some people like it with applesauce instead. I received this recipe attached to a gift of gingerbread mix in a jar, so many thanks to both the person who came up with the recipe and the person who gave it to me—my sister Deanna! As expected, I prefer to use whole wheat pastry flour for baking sweet treats.

Gingerbread

2½ cups flour

1½ teaspoons baking soda

½ teaspoon salt

1½ teaspoons ground ginger

1 teaspoon ground cinnamon

¼ **teaspoon ground clove**

½ **cup (1 stick) butter, softened**

1 **egg**

1 **cup old-fashioned molasses (do not use blackstrap molasses)**

1 **cup hot water**

Heat oven to 350 degrees. Grease and flour a 9-inch square baking pan. Sift the flour, soda, salt, ginger, cinnamon, and clove over a bowl. If you are making this for a gift, it will be easier to pour into the jar if you sift on a piece of waxed paper. Also, if you use the whole wheat pastry flour, there may be bits of bran left in the sifter—put them into the bowl too, just be sure there are no nuggets of salt or soda left.

In another bowl, cream the butter until soft, and then beat in the egg. Add the molasses and mix well. To this molasses mixture, add the flour mixture alternately with the hot water, stirring until well blended. Pour batter into prepared pan and bake for 30 minutes or until top springs back when lightly touched with your finger. Do not overbake. Cool in pan on wire rack. Cut into squares to serve.

A wonderful variation on this recipe can be achieved by adding ¼ cup chopped candied ginger to the dry ingredients (use your fingers to make sure the pieces don't stick together), and proceed as above.

To make a gift mix in a jar, simply pour the dry ingredients into a clean quart canning jar, top with the flat lid, then place a 6-inch square of calico or other homey fabric between the lid and ring (use pinking shears to cut the fabric for a nice effect), and use ribbon or twine to attach the complete recipe, which you have written on a suitable tag. I suppose you could just give the intended person a baked gingerbread, but this means they have to eat it on your schedule, which is the nice part about mix-in-a-jar gifts—they're ready when you are. They're also a good way to teach kids basic cooking techniques without too much fuss.

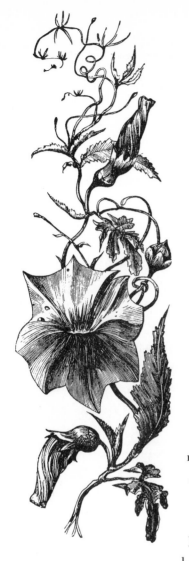

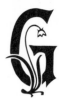

is for Grandma's
Magic Healing Salve

The basic technique for making salves, ointments, or unguents is discussed in "The Kitchen Apothecary" section beginning on page 3. However, since I have mentioned this very special concoction a few times throughout the book, I thought I would give it the place it deserves amongst the Home Remedies Hall of Fame. Grandma's magic healing salve is renowned for taking the ouch out of owies, putting the supple back into scabs, and returning the moisture into lips chapped by a week of steady wind across the phenomenal high desert of southern Oregon. Aw, heck—you can practically eat the stuff, it really is magic.

Get Personal

Really, I believe in this stuff so much that I create a ceremony for the harvesting of the herbs and the gathering of all the ingredients and equipment used to make the salve. In northern Idaho, this usually happens sometime in early June, when everything is up and reaching toward the sun. I gather the leaves and flowers of several plants and simmer them ever so gently in pure olive oil, strain the oil, and harden it with grated beeswax. It's very easy to make, and it is a good way to introduce young ones to the healing powers of common herbs and wild plants. They will also enjoy their own personal plant ceremony, should you choose to create one.

Be Positive

You will, of course, be able to make a positive identification of each plant you use, and show this to the children by cross-referencing with a well-illustrated field guide. My main rule with kids is that they should never eat anything without showing me first, preferably while the plant is still rooted and growing. Then I show them specific ways to identify the plant, show them a similar plant and how to distinguish the differences, and test them on it later. Most kids I've met have no problem eating and finding "wild food," or even harvesting herbs from the garden; it gives them a sense of purpose and satisfaction, and a knowledge that won't fade if we encourage their learning. When making grandma's magic healing salve, it's easy to appreciate a useful, aromatic concoction that is soothing to everyday scrapes and bruises and chapped lips, even if it *is* green (but it doesn't look green on your lips, I promise).

They're Really More like Guidelines

Here is a basic recipe for salve using a one-quart mini slow cooker, so you can get an idea of quantities needed for each ingredient. If you use a saucepan, just be sure to keep the heat at a bare simmer; you want to extract the healing compounds from the herbs, not cook them. Choose at least three different herbs from the list on page 148.

As is mentioned in "The Kitchen Apothecary," I like to use a mini slow cooker to infuse herbs in the oil. It's the perfect non-scorching type of heat, and the amount of herbs you can fit in it is enough to handle without concern for heaviness or gallons of warm green oil. If you don't want to use a slow cooker, just use a stainless steel or enameled saucepan and keep the heat low, way low (this method takes less time than the slow cooker).

How do you know when the oil is finished infusing? Start by looking at the color. It should be turning dark green, and the plant material itself should have lost some of its own green color. Some references say to cook the leaves until crisp, but I don't do it that way as it's almost burnt by that time and not as desirable, in my opinion.

. . . .

Grandma's Magic Healing Salve

3 cups chopped, shredded, or torn herb leaves or flowers

3 cups olive or almond oil (you may need a bit more to cover the herbs)

1–2 ounces grated beeswax

Combine the herbs and oil in slow cooker (or saucepan) and set it to low heat, uncovered, for 12 hours or overnight, stirring occasionally; add more oil if necessary to keep the herbs covered. When oil is colored dark green from the herbs, line a strainer with cheesecloth or some other material, set it into an appropriately sized saucepan, and pour the oil extract through the cloth and into the second pan. Squeeze as much oil out of the plant-stuff as possible before discarding it (it's too oily for the compost). Put the oil extract over low heat and add the grated beeswax, about 1 ounce wax to a pint of oil, and stir. You will have to experiment with the amount of wax, which is another good reason not to make too much at a time. Once the wax is fully dissolved, put a small spoonful of the oil-wax mixture onto a plate and wait for it to cool, then check for hardness. If it is to your liking, then carefully pour the oil blend into small shallow jars, lip balm pots, or what have you. Half-pint and quarter-pint wide-mouth canning jars are very practical for this purpose and easy to come by. The salve will shrink a bit as it cools, also becoming lighter in color. Do not cover until cool, and do not disturb the jars while cooling. If you are going to use this herbal oil for both salve and lip balm, pour some of the waxed oil into the larger jars first for salve, then take the rest and return to low heat to add a touch more wax to make the lip balm a little harder consistency. This salve is perfectly safe for dogs, cats, horses, and other farm animals in addition to humans. Grandma's magic healing salve makes a very nice gift. Makes approximately 3 cups.

Leaf and Flower

The following list is just that, a list. It does, however, reflect my personal priorities in what I like the most of in my salve, starting at the top. I will not tell you how much to use—that partly depends on what grows in your vicinity and the size of your simmering vessel. This is my usual list; you will create your own, and it will be just as magical.

- comfrey leaf
- heal-all (also known as self-heal) leaf and flower
- plantain leaf
- chickweed
- yarrow leaf and flower
- cedar leaves
- St. John's wort, flowering tops
- violet leaf
- rose petals
- mint leaves
- elderberry leaf
- sage leaves
- lavender leaves

- clover blossoms

- thyme sprigs

- rosemary leaf

- cinquefoil leaf

You will note that many of the culinary herbs, such as thyme, sage, and rosemary, have antiseptic properties and would be appropriate in this salve. Some people like to add cottonwood buds that they picked in late winter and kept in the freezer until now. We want the salve to be emollient as well, to lubricate and quench stressed skin, so flower petals and tender leaves such as chickweed and heal-all are part of the equation. I've even made purely flower petal salves, and they are fragrant and beautiful. I call it fairy flower butter, and it makes an exquisite lip balm. You can use rose petals, clover blossoms, calendula petals, monarda petals, lemon balm flowers, dandelion petals, hollyhocks, violets, and so on. This could be fun for an all-girl sleep-over—picking flowers in the afternoon and making the balm, the next day everyone taking some home.

Learn what healing plants grow where you live. These are the plants that grow where I live. Just be sure to properly identify, and you will be safe.

Who's Your Granny?

And that, too, is part of the magic—being a grandma, that is. It is a privilege and honor to be looked up to for guidance and comfort. At least it is for me. That, and a whole new generation I can get to listen to the Beatles!

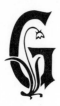

is for Gratitude —
*saying grace,
giving thanks*

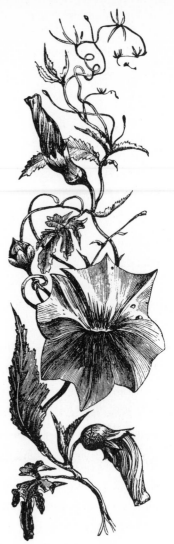

I get together with my circle
sisters once a month, when the
moon is full. We gather for a variety
of reasons, not the least of which is
to honor the earth mother and all of
creation. It is a spiritual gathering
as well as social, and we take turns
hostessing these events. After our
ceremony, we share a meal, but before
we eat, we gather hand in hand and say
a prayer to dedicate our feast to Creator,
Great Spirit, Goddess, God, Christos, Source (we are quite an eclectic
bunch). One way we honor Source is to fix a "spirit plate," onto which
is placed a small bit of all the foods we have brought to share. After
the dedication or meal blessing is spoken from the heart, we take the
plate outside and place it somewhere for the "spirits" to partake of.
(You might guess that some of these "spirits" turn out to be the furry,

four-legged domestic type, or sometimes even the wild or winged ones, but that doesn't matter. Who are we to dictate in what form Spirit will manifest?)

It's Nothing New

Every culture around the world, every spiritual inclination, every religious path has some form of thanks-giving for meals. Some are more elaborate than others; some take the form of days-long harvest feasts; but all are mindful of Mother Earth as provider of our sustenance. The plant kingdom as well as the animal kingdom is given a place of honor. Indeed, the symbiotic relationship of each to each is essential. Birds spread seeds from their droppings, cows and goats and other animals offer manure for fertilizing vegetable crops; I myself have gathered deer and moose droppings to mulch herb plants in my twenty-acre yard—don't laugh! One supplies the other in the cycle of life. Is it not perfect, the way everything is mutually supportive? What a beautiful pattern creation has woven for us.

There She Goes Again...

And then modern man somehow disrupts the equation. Valueless, nutritionless so-called "food" lines the shelves of the mega-markets. Oversalted (oh, my heart), overprocessed (devoid of life force), artificially flavored (flavor?) and colored (I'm sorry, but I've never seen a neon blue raspberry), junk junk junk! I have actually seen *microwavable* frozen organic dinners—like, what's the point of organic? Have we become a nation of spoiled, brain-dead pie holes bent on instant gratification, removed from how real food is created, removed from the source?

Okay, enough of the diatribe. Off the soapbox. No more proselytizing. We know what the problem is. How about a solution?

Time Out

The best way I can figure to overcome this sort of negativity is to give thanks for our food. Getting in touch with Source will create awareness not only in our minds but also in the minds of others, sort of like the pebble in the pond effect. The ripples spread out, touching other ripples, intersecting, creating new patterns.

Concerning the quality of modern food, I have a very creative friend who not only gives thanks for her meals, she also prays that her body extracts only what is beneficial to her and sheds what is unhealthy. Naturally, she tends to eat smart as a rule, but she doesn't cook a lot, eats out often, and is pretty healthy for someone in her mid-fifties. I think this is an interesting and valid method of thanks-giving.

When we give thanks, our hearts become full long before our bellies; a full heart is a happy heart. When we have the attitude of gratitude, many things become easier—sharing, giving, loving. It's part of us; I believe it's why we were created. Yes, I believe we were made to love.

How Can We Forget?

Remember to give thanks for your food, even if only in a silent, private way, even at a restaurant (so what if other people see you, maybe they'll get the idea). I guarantee it will make a difference in your life well beyond mealtime.

This is a simple prayer similar to what we might say before a meal:

Great Spirit Creator

Thank you for bringing us together to share this meal

Thank you for providing us with this good food and this good company

Truly, we are blessed

We ask that you bless others who may not be eating as well as us

And that you guide us safely throughout our journey

We thank you from the bottom of our heart

Ho!

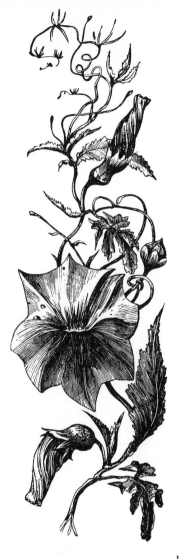

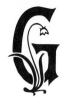

is for Greens
for Beans

No, this is not a recipe for a
vegetarian political party, it's a tasty,
tenderizing herbal blend added to a
simmering pot of beans. You can use
just about any kind of dry bean such
as pintos, navy or great northern, red
beans or kidney, even garbanzos, also
known as chickpeas. If you don't
have a local patch of nettles you
can harvest, purchase them at your
local natural food store, which is also
where you'll find the kelp. All the herbs
and spices called for in the recipe are dried, not fresh; try growing
some of these herbs at home and drying them yourself, you'll taste the
difference. This makes about 1½ cups seasoning blend and it takes 1
tablespoon herb blend to season a pot of beans.

· ·

Greens for Beans Seasoning Blend

½ cup chopped, crushed, or snipped kelp
(also known as kombu or konbu)

½ cup chopped nettle leaves

2 tablespoons garlic powder or granules
(do not use garlic salt)

2 tablespoons dried marjoram

2 tablespoons dried oregano

2 tablespoons dried sage

2 tablespoons savory

1 teaspoon ginger root powder

Combine all ingredients in a bowl, using your hands and fingers
to mix well, and store in a glass jar. Use 1 tablespoon blend for each
2 cups dry beans, which must first be washed and soaked overnight,
then thoroughly rinsed.

· ·

A Pot o' Beans

2 cups dry beans of your choice

1 tablespoon Greens for Beans herbal blend

2 teaspoons salt, or to taste

1–2 hot chilies, optional

Rinse beans and pick over for stones. In a large bowl, cover the
beans with plenty of water and soak overnight. The next day, drain
the beans and rinse thoroughly. In a large saucepan, cook beans in
double their volume of water or unsalted broth by first bringing to a
boil, boiling 10 minutes, then reducing the heat to a low simmer; skim
off any foam that accumulates. Then add the herbal blend. For a real
kicker, add 1 or 2 dried hot chilies as well. Simmer beans for 1 to 2
hours, uncovered, stirring occasionally, until beans are tender and no
longer starchy. Add more water if necessary to keep them covered. Do
not add salt until cooked through halfway, otherwise it will toughen

the beans (just don't forget the salt or the beans will taste flat). When the aroma fills the air, your meal companions will be surprised to find out it's "just a pot of beans." You can make a simple supper with these beans by baking corn or spice muffins and fixing a lemony coleslaw to accompany it.

If you want to use a slow cooker for the beans, just be sure to bring the beans to a boil in a separate pan for 10 minutes before putting them in the crock, then set on low and away you go. You'll just have to add the salt later.

It's important to soak the beans overnight in plenty of water with lots of rinsing afterward to remove certain saccharides, which cause gas. It's also important to boil the beans for 10 minutes before setting them on a simmer so they don't ferment before they're hot enough, which makes them difficult to digest and causes more gas and bloating. Even so, some people cannot eat beans no matter how they are prepared.

The kelp also helps tenderize the bean and is used extensively in macrobiotic cooking. You can buy kelp—which is a type of seaweed, usually *Laminaria* spp.—as powder or granules, but I prefer to use the dried, leafy sheets and chop it up myself. It's a chore, but it's less gritty too. What I do is cut the kelp up into tiny ribbons with sharp kitchen shears. Be sure to use food-grade kelp and not kelp processed for garden amendment. Kelp is also made into very thin sheets called *nori*, which is used to wrap sushi rolls.

Incidentally, I use nettle leaf in this recipe as compared to nettle herb, which includes the stem as well; this is okay for beverage teas or soup broths that you strain, but it's not as enjoyable floating around in a bowl of beans. For more ways to use nettles, see page 219, "N is for Nettles."

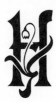

is for Hawthorn—
a shrub? a tree?

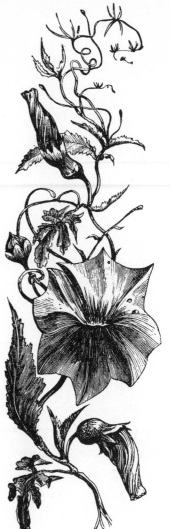

Although the hawthorn tree usually grows like a large shrub, here in northern Idaho there are huge treelike specimens on the islands in the river near my home. Back in 1976, the state champion down near the Clearwater River had a circumference of 64 inches, which is quite large for a shrubby tree. Hawthorns have one- to two-inch thorns that like to ferociously reach out and grab you, pulling at your hair and tearing holes in your sleeves; similar to blackberries, the wild fruit is not necessarily free for the picking. Belonging to the vast Rosaceae, or rose, family, this shrubby tree of the temperate zone is cold hardy and a good bird tree, with many ornamental varieties available to the home gardener. The fruit has been used to make jam and liqueur, and the wood is so dense that charcoal made from it is supposed to burn hot enough to use in a smithy's forge.

Way Back When

The fruit is called haws, from an Old Saxon word meaning "hedge," and refers to early hedge plantings of hawthorn common in medieval Britain; perhaps this is what Prince Charming had to hack his way through to rescue Sleeping Beauty from her fairy-tale coma. Some early Christians believed this tree to be the crown of thorns placed on the head of Jesus at the crucifixion, but this is unlikely because hawthorns did not grow in the Middle East. Perhaps because of this association, some folks during the Middle Ages believed that bringing hawthorn into the home would cause a family member to die. In her book *Common Herbs for Natural Health*, herbalist and world traveler Juliette de Bairacli Levy says that European Gypsies gathered hawthorn to encourage the fey folk to visit. Celtic legend relates that where the triad of oak, ash, and thorn grow together, one may see the faeries. Hawthorn has been associated with the sixth moon cycle of the year, which is one reason why it is also called May. (Remember that while there may only be twelve calendar months to a year, there are thirteen lunations, or moon cycles.) On May Day, or Beltane as it is sometimes called, the Cornish folk would deck their doorways with flowering branches of hawthorn to herald spring. An old beauty charm instructs us to wash in the dew of hawthorn blossoms at dawn on May Day to make us "ever after handsome be." Hey, it couldn't hoit!

The Heart of the Matter

What better way to encourage good looks than to encourage good health? The magic of the hawthorn is that it is a very gentle nervine, but most notably, hawthorn is a subtle heart tonic, strengthening weak conditions and easing excessive conditions. It mildly dilates the blood vessels and lowers blood pressure. Hawthorn does not have a direct effect on the heart but rather a gradual toning of the heart muscle, with the bonus of increasing oxygen utilization. And while it doesn't alter heart disease, there are no negative side effects from using it. However, if you are already taking medications for your heart and you want to consider using hawthorn, please check with your physician first, although it is unlikely that he or she will know anything about it.

For sheer enjoyment, consider sipping a tasty tonic decoction of roots & fruits tea (see "T is for Tea," page 265, for the recipe), especially in early spring. Bring 1 pint of water to a boil, add 2 heaping teaspoons herbal tea blend (or plain dried hawthorn berries), reduce heat to a simmer and cover, steeping for about 10 minutes; strain and serve, sweetened with honey if desired. In addition to this nonmedicinal tea, you can also make hawthorn tincture or extract (see page 10 of "The Kitchen Apothecary" for instructions on how to make a tincture). The parts to harvest are the white or pinkish flowers in the spring, including the woody little branch-stem to which it is attached (it's okay if there is a leaf on the stem), and tincture these fresh. Then, in late summer, harvest the purplish black berries, or "haws," and tincture those too, separately. When each has steeped for the appropriate time (usually 2 to 4 weeks), combine the two extracts for a compound tincture of hawthorn flowers and fruit. This is what I do for myself as a preventative, since heart disease and high cholesterol runs in my dad's family and I like butter and cheese. The choline content in hawthorn helps break up fat into tiny molecules so it passes through arterial tissues easier and reduces the buildup of cholesterol in the arteries.

Spiritual Medicine

I have made it clear throughout this book that I am not a medical herbalist, but I wanted to include the information about hawthorn and the heart because it is very mild and slow-acting, and is not directly medicinal, like foxglove, for instance, and its well-known drug derivative, digitalis. As a simple beverage tea, hawthorn probably won't affect the heart at all except to tone and normalize it, and even this occurs only after using it regularly over several weeks' time. In other words, it's very safe.

Hawthorn berry tea also tastes good, which is reason enough to drink it, and who couldn't use a good tonic in the spring? Plus, I think me and She have a special rapport, a sort of mutual communion. Sipping tea in the early morning, spying robins as they listen for grubs and worms, catching the sun's warm fingers peeking over the ridge — all are good medicine for the heart. It's a peaceful time of day, perfect for contemplation. The branches of the hawthorn tree are a good place to leave prayer ties. Just don't be surprised if Granny Whitethorn decides to snag a piece of your shirt for her own tie.

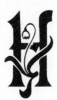

is for Honey Cakes—
two kinds

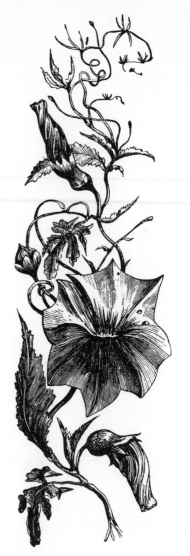

Both these cakes are delicious. I love recipes that feature honey as the sweetener. You can use unbleached all-purpose flour or, my preference, whole wheat pastry flour in either of these recipes; you might use just a touch less if using the whole wheat.

. . . .

Honey Pound Cake

½ cup (1 stick) butter, softened

¾ cup honey

3 eggs, slightly beaten

1 teaspoon vanilla extract

2 cups flour

2½ teaspoons baking powder

½ teaspoon salt

¼ teaspoon baking soda

½ cup milk

Grease and flour a bread loaf pan. Preheat oven to 350 degrees. Beat the butter until creamy; add honey and beat until fluffy. Next, add the eggs and vanilla, beating again until well blended.

Stir flour, baking powder, salt, and baking soda in a separate bowl. Alternating between flour mixture and milk, add each to honey butter, blending well after each addition. Pour batter into prepared pan and smooth evenly.

Bake about 45 minutes, or until loaf tests done with a wooden pick. Cool in pan 10 minutes, and then turn onto rack to cool thoroughly. Wrap airtight and store at room temperature for 8 hours before slicing.

Makes 1 loaf cake.

. . . .

Joyful Honey Carrot Cake

1 cup honey

1 cup oil, such as sunflower

4 eggs

2 cups flour

1 teaspoon baking powder

1 teaspoon baking soda

¼ teaspoon salt

1 teaspoon ground cinnamon

½ teaspoon ground cardamom

½ teaspoon ginger root powder

3 cups grated carrot (about 6 or 7 carrots,
    or approximately 1 pound)

1 cup sunflower seeds (pecans are good too)

½ cup raisins (or currants)

Grease and flour a 9 by 13-inch glass baking dish. Preheat oven to 350 degrees.

Beat the honey, oil, and eggs together in one bowl, mixing well. In a separate bowl, stir flour, baking powder, baking soda, salt, cinnamon, cardamom, and ginger together, and then add to honey mixture.

Finally, stir in the carrots, sunflower seeds, and raisins so all are well distributed. Spread into prepared pan. Bake for 35 to 40 minutes, or until cake tests done with a wooden pick. Top with cream cheese spread (below), if desired.

Makes 1 large cake.

. . . .

Cream Cheese Spread

Soften 1 (8-ounce) package cream cheese and mix with ¼ cup honey, blending well; spread on cooled cake and cut into squares to serve.

Honey On the Body, As Well As In

In addition to using honey in treats such as these cakes, honey also has a place in the kitchen apothecary. Honey is antimicrobial and bacteria will not grow in it, so it can be spread on minor wounds and scrapes, and most notably on burns. You can use honey as a facial while you relax in a warm tub—just tie your hair back and spread the sticky, sweet amber all over your face and neck and settle in; simply wash it off in the water after you've had enough.

There's a Time and a Place

One special and important note about honey here. I have mentioned several times throughout this book not to give honey to babies under a year old. The reason for this is that while bacteria does not grow in honey, the bacteria *Clostridium botulinum* (the one that causes botulism toxicity) produces spores that are very heat resistant, and these spores can sometimes be found in honey, especially raw honey. While I totally advocate using raw honey that hasn't had all the healthful enzymes cooked out of it (and when making herbal syrups, you'll notice my instruction to heat at a very low temperature), and while these spores are not harmful to the healthy human adult body, they may possibly cause an infection in the infant's intestinal tract. Therefore, honey should not be fed to infants, even in cooked foods. They don't need sweets anyway.

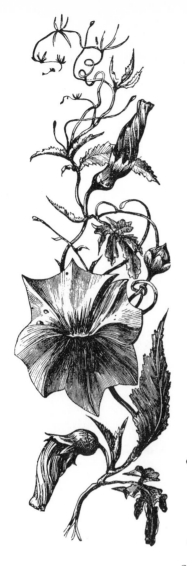

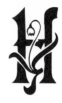

is for Horseradish

Even though horseradish was unknown to the ancient Hebrews, modern Jews often use it as one of the five bitter herbs during the Passover feast. These herbs symbolize the suffering experienced during captivity in Egypt; the Passover celebrates the time when the god of the Israelites passed them over, smiting their captors instead. The five herbs are horseradish, nettle, coriander, horehound, and lettuce (some say chicory). I think maybe they use it because it goes good with pot roast.

Best eaten fresh, horseradish is used grated as a pungent and nasally existential condiment, producing a kind of orgasm to the sinuses—oh, yes, I love it! Horseradish is excellent with roast beef or any other roasted red meat. It is also a nice surprise in creamy mashed potatoes. Horseradish is a perfect appetite stimulant and liver tonic to accompany these rich foods.

. . . .

Fresh Preserved Horseradish

½ cup peeled, finely grated horseradish

½ teaspoon salt

3–4 tablespoons white wine vinegar

Simply combine all the ingredients and spoon into a small jar. If necessary, use another spoonful of vinegar in order to cover the horseradish completely. This concoction will keep for a couple weeks refrigerated. You could also use bottled lemon juice as a variation (like vinegar, bottled juice has a specific pH, or constant acidity, useful when preserving food). If you want to mix it with sour cream to make horseradish sauce, squeeze out the vinegar as much as possible (and perhaps use it for your salad).

You can also make horseradish syrup for mucous-producing coughs and bronchitis. See page 14 of "The Kitchen Apothecary" for instructions on how to make herbal syrups.

If you want to grow a horseradish plant, keep in mind that it is quite large at two to three feet tall and that the gophers at my place just love it. Last year we planted some in a fifteen-gallon pot, which we sunk into the ground for moisture retention and to gopher-proof the root. We finally harvested it this spring to use the root and replant the massive crown (we had to break it up into four pieces, actually). The root itself was also massive and tastes great. One of the big debates about horseradish is whether to harvest in spring or fall. Try it and see for yourself.

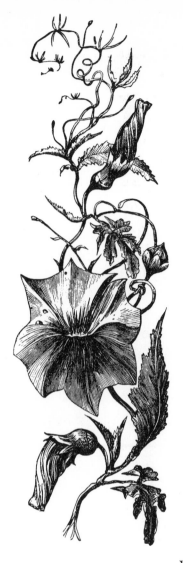

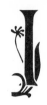

is for Insect
Repellents —
*natural ways
to bug off!*

Ahh,   summer ... hiking,
swimming, picnics ... and visitors,
most of whom we welcome with open
arms. Some visitors, however, become
pests, and insects are among them.
Rather than using toxic sprays or
powders to repel bugs or kill them,
we can use herbs to repel them instead.
Whether wild or cultivated, these
insect-repelling herbs are much cheaper
and safer (as long as you don't eat them) than store-bought. Please note
that pregnant women shouldn't handle most of these herbs (especially
tansy, mugwort, and pennyroyal), as they can be very potent, even
through the skin. The lavender spray described below is one exception,
however, and can be safely sprayed on clothing and hats and such.

Tansy

Some herbs are effective for keeping bugs away from animals too. One of the most common wild plants used for repelling insects is tansy. It is easy to identify and collect and usually grows prolifically; it also dries nicely for floral arrangements. Hung in bunches near doorways, windows, in and around animal stalls and barns, it is used as a fly repellent. Be sure to keep it where the animals can't eat it, because it is toxic in large amounts—same for humans: don't eat it! To repel ants, sprinkle dried and crumbled tansy flower and leaf around house foundations, thresholds, cupboards, and anywhere in their path.

Moth Repellents

Tansy is also a moth-repelling herb, as are rosemary, wormwood, lavender, citrus peel, aromatic cedar, spearmint, and patchouli. You can use a single herb of your choice or make pleasing combinations and tie them into little cloth bags to lie amongst linens, woolens, in the blanket chest, or from hangers in the closet. It's what you might call a potpourri with a purpose.

Flies and Other Vermin

Peppermint and pennyroyal can be hung in bunches to ward off flies, and they have also been dried, crumbled, and used like tansy to keep away ants and mice. Cats can also help keep mice away (well, some do); to keep fleas from bugging the cats, make a small cloth collar and fill with pennyroyal, citrus peel, and eucalyptus. These herbs can be stuffed in a bed pillow for cats or dogs, with a lofty base of aromatic cedar shavings. Many herbalists suggest rubbing pennyroyal oil behind the ears of your pet where they can't lick it off, and this method does work well, but the distilled oil is very dangerous if used around pregnant women, so I recommend using the cloth collar filled with herbs instead. Do not use this collar or the oil on your pet if they are pregnant.

Mosquitoes

For mosquitoes and no-see-ums, a handful of any of these fresh herbs crushed and then rubbed on arms, legs, hats, etc., makes an effective yet fragrant repellent: pennyroyal, tansy (okay, not so fragrant), basil, lavender, marigold (the common border plant), thyme, or yarrow (I love the smell of yarrow). If you are bitten, crush a plantain leaf into a pulp (you can just chew it up a little), then put the pulp on the bite; relief should be immediate. (See page 234, "P is for Plantain," for other uses of this common weed.) Citronella candles placed around the room or outdoor sitting area also make a good mosquito repellent. These are very easy to make with the essential oil added to the wax. For pregnant women, a lavender insect-repelling spray (see below) would be a safe choice.

. . . .

Insect-Repelling Spray

Steep 1 ounce dried lavender or other herbs of choice in 1 pint rubbing alcohol or preferably 100-proof vodka for 7 to 10 days; strain, then pour to halfway in a spray bottle and fill the rest of the way with water. Carefully label. Keep the remaining solution in a glass bottle until needed. Under no circumstances should this liquid be ingested. Spray or apply frequently as an insect repellent—don't inhale the spray, and avoid your eyes. You can spray it on hats and shirts too.

Here's an even easier version that takes less than a minute to prepare: Simply fill your spray bottle with common prepared witch hazel and add several drops lemon-eucalyptus essential oil, close the container, and shake well. Label and spray away. This is supposed to be as effective as low levels of deet, which we *definitely* want to avoid. And it's lemon-eucalyptus, not lemon and eucalyptus, essential oil. You could alternatively use lavender essential oil, especially for pregnant women.

On a hot day, the cooling alcohol and green herbal scent can be fairly pleasant. Vinegar can be used instead of alcohol, but the smell is, well ... I guess there are worse things than smelling like a salad. But it just might work in getting rid of those *other* visitors who've overstayed their welcome!

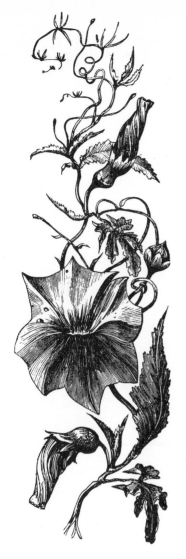

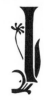 is for Italian
Herban Tomatoes—
the "H" is silent,
Martha

Many thanks to my old friend
Coyote Woman for this utterly
delicious, height-of-summertime
delight. This salad practically vibrates
with goodness. The original recipe
called for sliced scallion; I prefer
minced red onion or shallot, and I
suggest that you use what you prefer
or, more importantly, what is fresh and
available. It is very easy to prepare. No
measured amounts are given here—use your own taste, as judicious or
as lavish as you wish. Let the tomatoes marinate for at least one hour
before serving.

· ·

Italian Herban Tomatoes

COMBINE:

Sliced vine-ripened tomatoes (hit the farmer's market early)

Minced red onion or shallot, or sliced scallions

Minced fresh garlic

Fresh chopped parsley

SEASON WITH:

Oregano, fresh if available

Salt and pepper

Pinch of sugar

Olive oil

Red wine vinegar

These tomatoes are fabulous served with crusty bread and grilled anything, or just the bread...and may the nectar of the Mountain Goddess fill your chalice!

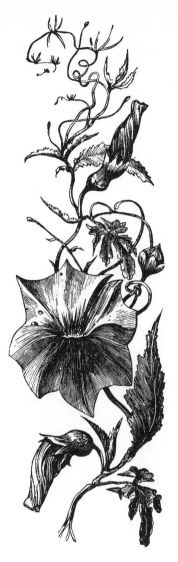

is for Java—
cookies with caffeine!

Jumpin' jiminy! Here are three
recipes for cookies that feature coffee
as a flavoring. One is an easy-to-
make bar cookie, the other keeps very
well for the holidays, and the third
is a rich shortbread made of dreams.
I recommend a medium-roast coffee
for these recipes rather than a dark
French or espresso roast, although
you will want the coffee grounds
powdery fine.

. . . .

Coffee Nut Bars with Chocolate Chips

½ cup (1 stick) butter, softened

¾ cup brown sugar

1 egg

½ teaspoon vanilla extract

1 cup flour (whole wheat pastry flour is my preference)

1 tablespoon fresh ground coffee, powdery fine grind

½ teaspoon baking soda

½ teaspoon salt

1 cup pecans

1 cup semi-sweet chocolate chips

Cream butter and sugar thoroughly. Add egg and vanilla, blending well. In a separate bowl, stir the flour, coffee, baking soda, and salt together, and add to butter mixture, mixing until all is incorporated. Add pecans and chocolate chips (try using white chocolate chips for variety). Spread batter into a greased 8 by 8-inch square baking pan. Bake at 350 degrees for about 35 minutes—do not overbake. Cool and cut into squares. Makes 1 pan.

The next recipe derives its name from the German for "pepper nuts." My aunt Valerie gave me the recipe many years ago. She makes them early in November so the flavors can meld and so they're ready for Christmas. Dunk into steaming hot java on a cold winter morning and let the spices warm you from the inside out. This recipe makes a whopping 18 dozen, but it can be halved easily.

. . . .

Pfefferneusse

1 cup dark corn syrup

1 cup honey

1 cup (2 sticks) butter, softened

1½ cups sugar

3 eggs

3 teaspoons baking soda

¾ cup cold strong brewed coffee

1 teaspoon ground black pepper

1 tablespoon whole aniseed

2 teaspoons ground cinnamon

½ teaspoon salt

10–11 cups sifted flour (I prefer whole
   wheat pastry flour, unsifted)

Powdered sugar for dusting

First, place the corn syrup, honey, butter, sugar, eggs, and baking soda in a very large bowl. Beat until well blended; an electric mixer helps, if you have one.

Next, mix in the coffee, black pepper, aniseed, cinnamon, salt, and half the flour. Stir in enough of the remaining flour to make a stiff— "but not crumbly," says Aunt Val—dough. You will need a bit of elbow grease for this. Cover the cookie dough and refrigerate overnight. Next day, shape dough into walnut-sized balls. Place on an ungreased baking sheet an inch or two apart (they don't spread much), and bake in a preheated 350-degree oven for 12 to 15 minutes. Place on wire rack and immediately dust with powdered sugar. Cool completely, then store in an airtight container to mellow for several weeks.

The following recipe was a special request given to me courtesy of Lulu's Confections. It is easy to make and easier to devour. Lulu delivers her cookies by bicycle in Portland, Oregon. Lulu sez, "Eat them alone, or share them with friends. Impress the girl or boy in your life." Shouldn't be a problem.

. . . .

Caffe Shortbread

10 tablespoons butter (1 stick plus 2 tablespoons)

½ cup sugar

½ teaspoon vanilla extract

Pinch salt

1¼ cups all-purpose flour

1 tablespoon finely ground coffee
(powdery fine, as for espresso)

Mix the butter, sugar, and salt together, either in a mixer or with a fork. Blend well, but don't overdo it—shortbread doesn't like a lot of extra air. Mix in the flour and ground coffee until it gets a crumbly, pealike texture.

Preheat oven to 300 degrees. Using a rolling pin dusted with a bit of flour (and dusting the table as well), get to rolling. Turn the dough as you go so it doesn't stick. It might be helpful to roll out the dough on a sheet of waxed paper. Make it a half-inch thick or so—shortbread is fat. Cut shapes with a cookie cutter, a glass, or a knife. Using a spatula, carefully place on an ungreased baking sheet. Bake for about 25 minutes. Do not rush the baking by turning the temperature up; it will ruin the cookies.

Recipe note: One tester recommended using powdered (confectioner's) sugar in the recipe and chilling the dough in a flattened disc (such as for pie dough) for an hour before rolling and cutting. They also suggest lining the baking sheet with parchment paper and baking for 8 to 10 minutes at 325 degrees. There are many factors that can affect the results of any given recipe, especially baked goods, such as elevation, humidity, flour, butter (some brands are more "liquidy" than others), and so on. Where you live will also affect results.

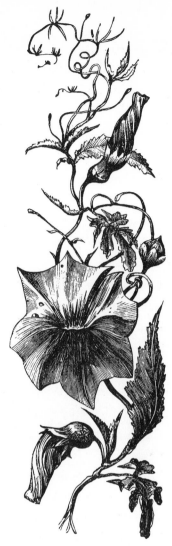

is for the Journey
to the Center of
Your Mind—
*or, meetings with
remarkable plant
spirits*

Plant spirits? Am I out of my airy-fairy Aquarian mind? What are plant spirits, and what do they have to do with you and me?

Throughout many cultures, there is a primordial belief in the spirit of plants, a numinous animation that may be intuited or felt in ways difficult to explain. Shamans and medicine workers are known to enter into a deep meditative state to visit the spirit world and return with just the right "medicine," or plant remedy, to treat their patron. The shaman meets the spirit of the plant on his or her "journey," and the plant spirit gives him or her instructions on how to use it. Sometimes the plant is not ingested but is used in other ways according to the information received by the shaman or medicine healer.

We may wonder what this animistic practice has to do with us here and now, in the age of wireless communication and the exchange and collection of information via satellite. While the dictionary may define animism as a primitive belief system, practitioners of a technique called journeying will tell you that communicating with plant spirits is a very relevant and useful form of information gathering. Journeying is not used for calling up ghosts or the spirits of dead people, and it is nothing like a séance. It is a tool for understanding the self and for finding ways of helping others. Similar to the dream state (see page 294, "X is for Xanadu"), the experiences you have or entities you encounter during a journey are very personal and individualized, yet the messages they give may be applied to the community at large.

Perhaps one of the most renowned explorations of human-plant communication in our era is that of the Findhorn Community in northern Scotland and its co-founder Dorothy MacLean. A secretary with British Intelligence who worked in offices and embassies worldwide, MacLean was a religious woman with a deep, abiding faith. She began to spontaneously hear voices and, encouraged by her studies of metaphysics (and in spite of some of her friends thinking she was loony), decided to start listening to what the voices had to say. MacLean eventually met Peter and Eileen Caddy through her Sufi teacher. Parents of three active boys, Peter was a former RAF official and mountain climber, and Eileen was a busy mother and spiritual clairvoyant. The three of them formed a friendship and went to work together at a country inn. After six years of working there, they were all let go. Mind you, all this initially took place in the late 1950s, in a very religiously conservative Great Britain. Following prompts received during meditation and desperate for shelter before the coming winter, they ended up in a caravan (camping trailer) on the beach near Findhorn, and the following spring they attempted to grow vegetables in the brackish, sandy soil. Needless to say, it wasn't going all that well at first, but the friends continued to follow their spiritual inclinations, which included remaining receptive to the voices.

And then one day, it happened: Dorothy was greeted by a Pea Deva, as she called it (*deva* meaning "being of light" in Hindi). In *The Magic of Findhorn*, author Paul Hawken says that this being was "certainly not a pea. It was something that moved through and around the materiality that was a garden pea." MacLean realized that she was not communicating with the spirit of an individual pea plant but "a spirit which was the plan, the mold, and architect of all the peas on earth."

Other plant devas began to communicate with MacLean (she got to know quite a few of them), at first with purely practical information. This resulted in the flourishing of the very garden where she first encountered them. Locals would come by the caravan park to gawk at the fabulous veggies produced on the blustery Scottish coastline. Later, when there was more than enough to feed the family (and to generate some income), the gardeners began selling their miraculous vegetables. One of the amendments they used in their garden was seaweed, gathered from the cove where they camped and applied as mulch; they also scrounged old produce from the local market and manure from a neighboring horse pasture to make compost, something from which we could all take a lesson.

The plant devas eventually communicated information of a more universal nature, that of brotherhood and environmental awareness. The attention MacLean and the Caddys received and the subsequent Findhorn community phenomenon is a continuing story in the transcendental relationship between humans and the world unseen.

There are a number of studies documented in the now-classic *The Secret Life of Plants* by Peter Tompkins and Christopher Bird, and some of these describe how common houseplants were wired with sensors to record the plant's physical changes in response to environmental changes and, more interestingly, human attitude and intention toward the plants. I remember reading this book as a teen (I guess that makes me a classic, too) and feeling validated for all those conversations I had with the trees, grasses, and flowers—kind of freaky!

Along these same lines—and certainly no less phenomenal, if not controversial—is the gathering and use of what are called flower essences. These are not essential oils, nor are they fragrant aromas. Flower essences, or perhaps more correctly flower essence remedies, are produced by gathering specific flowers on a sunny, cloudless day, depositing them into glass bowls of purified water, and steeping them for a few hours to absorb the essence of the flower; they are further diluted until the proper dosage strength is achieved and preserved with a drop of brandy. Unlike homeopathic remedies, which are basically highly diluted tinctures (alcohol-plant extracts) used to stimulate the body's own healing response, flower essences don't contain any of the plant's molecules at all. Flower essences are not extracts, they are energetic potions, and there is admittedly a tremendous leap of faith in using these remedies, but anyone who's tried Rescue Remedy is likely a believer. Their purpose is to impart emotional and spiritual healing and beneficence to the user. The flower itself tells the practitioner how to use it, and remedies are chosen intuitively; two or three essences may be combined to make a personalized remedy.

And how does one come to realize which flower is useful for which condition? By talking to the plants, of course!

There are several terms used for human-plant communication, and one is called attunement—we are attempting to "tune in" to the spirit or indwelling entity of the plant. And while this type of meditative exercise may be shamanic in approach, you do not have to be a shaman or healing practitioner of any sort to communicate with plants. The biggest prerequisite for this intuitive approach is an open heart and mind and a willingness to allow for the possibility. It is perfectly acceptable to bring along a healthy dose of skepticism; after all, even in the wizarding world (according to *Harry Potter and the Chamber of Secrets*), hearing voices is not "normal." But who said anything about being normal?

Recipe for Plant-Spirit Communication

To begin, first decide on the plant with whom you want to communicate. It can be a houseplant such as an aloe vera or Swedish ivy or an outdoor plant such as a wild strawberry or daffodil. Do not pick the plant; leave it in the soil. Bring along a pen and pad of paper. Find a quiet place near the plant, seat yourself comfortably, and do what you can to avoid interruptions. Close your eyes and take three slow, deep breaths. Inform the plant of your intention (which at this point is simply to communicate with it). Make an offering to the plant—many Native American practitioners use tobacco, but you could use cornmeal, a snippet of your hair, or even bit of nourishing compost—and sprinkle it at the base of the plant. Intention is the most important factor.

Now, sit quietly and simply observe. Look at the plant with "fuzzy vision" (or "soft eyes," as my yoga teacher would say), trace your finger along the veins, feel the delicate leaves, allow yourself to merge with the textures and subtleties of the plant. You are not trying to see with your eyes, you are trying to see with your intuition. Allow your mind to open and let the stream of consciousness flow. Take as much time as you need. Then, with pen and paper, record any words, feelings, or emotions that come to you, no matter how strange or insignificant they may seem at first. Perhaps there will be music involved, or other sounds, or colors or textures. Write it down or draw it.

Tell the plant who you are and how much you appreciate it. Let it know how it beautifies your life and that you wish to know it better. The next step is to listen. Listen with your heart for any type of energetic response. You can keep your eyes open or closed. Listen quietly. Do not judge what you experience, just keep a note of it. You can decipher the messages later.

If you don't receive a recognizable response, don't worry. And don't give up after your first attempt. Thank the plant again and bid it farewell for the time being, knowing that you can revisit it again in the future, and perhaps it will be more communicative and you will be more receptive. There is no wrong way to communicate with plant-spirits unless you knowingly disrespect them or the plants. If you approach the process with love and respect, no harm will be done.

Once you have practiced plant-spirit attunement and become more adept at this form of wireless communication, you will be ready for the next step, which is journeying to the spirit world to find your animal guardian and medicine plant. This is assuming that your interest in communicating with plant spirits blooms into sharing the information with others for the benefit of all. Medicine workers and shamans do not do this sort of work for their own amusement; they do it for the good of the people. However, there is nothing wrong with visiting plant spirits for personal self-improvement.

My own experience with plant-spirit communication is pretty narrow. However, the experiences were enlightening and amazing. You may wonder if the messages received are made up, if they are what you wanted to hear in the first place. All I can say is that you have to experience it for yourself; we cannot see the wind, yet we can see the result of it. So I'll go out on a limb here like another well-known MacLaine and say that I believe in plant spirits and other-dimensional beings because I have experienced them. Here are notes from my plant-spirit journey to cottonwood; this is what it told me:

> The balm of me is in your hands. Use my balm/your hands to send me energetically. I am so common, so common, [and] I'm special in that I'm a survivor. Just look at me: I have scars all over, yet I survive. Use me, my balm, on the knees, shoulders, stiff joints. Use my fragrant balm to send to people the essence of survival and overcoming injuries.

Then the cottonwood spirit had me draw hands with leaves coming out of the fingers, to emphasize the part about using "my balm/your hands" for healing. Indeed, the salve or balm made from unopened cottonwood buds is soothing to sore muscles, antiseptic on the skin (bees use the resin to make propolis, and propolis was also one of the ingredients used to embalm Egyptian mummies), and cottonwood oil is incredibly fragrant. My journey to the plant-spirit of yerba buena (*Satureja douglasii*) was more vague, although I did get the message that it was okay to talk to it but it wasn't into communicating at that time. C'est la vie.

I hope this introduction to the unseen world of plant spirits has intrigued you enough to at least give it some thought. The concept is as old as humanity, and while the early church discouraged people from practicing their folkways and the lords of the Age of Reason categorized and calculated everything within their clutches, science has finally caught up with magic and determined that inanimate objects have an energy field. If a rock has an aura, it doesn't take much imagination to suppose that plants and trees and flowers have some sort of animating spirit. It makes taking a nap leaned up against the old oak tree a whole new experience.

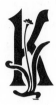

is for Kasha—
don't pass on the buckwheat, please

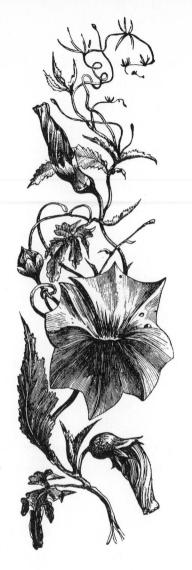

Kasha is so important to Slavic cultural identity that there are several metaphorical expressions referring to it in the Russian language. For instance, if you can't make kasha with a person, you won't get anywhere with them; and can you imagine Led Zeppelin's memorable song going something like "I've had kasha in my head for so long it's not true"?

Kasha is a common staple food served in most eastern European and Russian kitchens and is made from buckwheat (*Polygonum fagopyrum*). While we may think of buckwheat as a cereal, it is not a true grain even though it is sometimes referred to as buckwheat groats, which means "grain"—go figure. Botanically, it is related to rhubarb. This native of northern and central Asia is said to withstand harsh climates and will ripen even in poor soil. In farming, it is used extensively as a green (live-growing) manure and is well known as a bee plant—buckwheat honey is quite distinctive. And who doesn't love the hearty taste of buckwheat pancakes with sweet maple syrup? (Don't ask my husband!) There are several cultivars of buckwheat, as well as several wild cousins.

Japanese cooks are no stranger to buckwheat either; they have been turning it into soba, or buckwheat noodles, for centuries. Soba noodles are specially eaten on the Japanese New Year for prosperity in the coming year; all grains are connected with abundance in one way or another. According to macrobiotic theory, this somewhat triangular-shaped kernel is said to provide the body with a reservoir of energy and stamina, especially in the fall and winter. Buckwheat is a source of rutin, a bioflavonoid that contributes to capillary strength.

The word *kasha* did not always specifically refer to buckwheat. This term was brought to the United States by Jewish immigrants around the beginning of the twentieth century. Similar to the word *corn* in Great Britain, it referred to other grains as well, such as an oat kasha for breakfast. Hundreds of years ago, the word also meant "feast," with tales of splendid kashas given by magnanimous rulers. Kasha was an important ritual food, a fundamental component of weddings, funerals, and even peace-treaty signings.

I hope it doesn't require détente for you to try the following dish. Some versions of the recipe tell you to mix the egg and buckwheat right in the skillet; I like it better stirring it up in a bowl first. This recipe makes 4 servings as a side dish.

. . . .

Kasha

> 1 cup buckwheat
>
> 1 egg, slightly beaten
>
> 2 cups boiling hot chicken broth or water
>
> 2 tablespoons butter
>
> Salt and pepper

Start by heating a large, heavy skillet over medium heat. Stir buckwheat and egg together in a bowl. Pour into skillet and stir until the grains are separate and dry; the egg may stick a bit at first. Add the broth or water, butter, and seasonings, stirring one more time. Cover tightly and lower heat to a simmer, as for rice. Check after 15 minutes for doneness (it should remain a little chewy) and drain excess liquid if necessary; do not let the kasha get mushy.

There are many varieties of the basic kasha recipe. Some feature wild mushrooms, another important staple of the eastern European kitchen. Some use kasha as a filling for piroshki, a sort of vegetable pastry or Slavic potsticker. There is even dessert kasha with nuts, dried fruit, and spices. Once you know how to make the basic recipe, you can experiment to suit your own taste.

You can take the kasha recipe one step further (well, two), and imagine your own Jewish grandma cooking this next meal just for you.

Kasha Varnishke

Make one recipe basic kasha, as instructed above. While it's simmering, sauté 1 medium onion in about 1 teaspoon schmaltz (rendered chicken fat) or butter; keep warm. Meanwhile, boil 1 cup bow-tie pasta in plenty of salted water until done to your liking, or about 12 minutes. In a large bowl, combine the hot kasha with the onions and pasta, salt to taste, and serve.

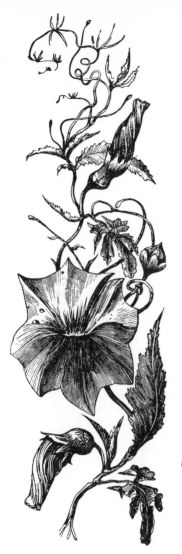

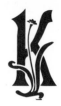

is for Kooka's Kalooa

Perhaps I should name this "coffee liqueur," but I don't think anyone will mind. No matter what it's called, this is the way I make it. Kalooa makes a most welcome gift. The recipe makes a little over a gallon—four bottles for giveaway and a bit for yourself.

. . . .

Kalooa

FOR THE COFFEE:

**1 pound medium-grind coffee (don't use
French roast or espresso)**

2 quarts water

FOR THE SUGAR SYRUP:

4 to 6 cups sugar, according to your sweet tooth

2 quarts water

2 ounces vanilla extract or 1 vanilla bean, split in half

FOR THE LIQUOR:

1 fifth (750 ml) brandy

1 fifth (750 ml) rum, preferably gold

Have ready two clean 1-gallon jars; you will use one for steeping, and you might need the other for mixing back and forth.

For the coffee, bring the water to a boil in a large saucepan, and add the coffee. Turn the heat way down and simmer, uncovered, about 20 minutes, stirring occasionally. Let cool for a few minutes. Into another saucepan, strain the brewed coffee through a sieve lined with a wet cloth—this could take a while, so be patient. There probably won't be 2 quarts now, since the coffee grounds have absorbed some of the water.

Next, stir the sugar and water in a saucepan, and simmer for just a few minutes, until the sugar is dissolved. Cool to lukewarm. Add whichever form of vanilla you choose.

Pour the cooled coffee into a gallon jar. Pour the vanilla syrup and the rum and brandy into the same jar. If there is too much to fit into one gallon jar, you'll have to divide it into two jars.

Cover the jar with waxed paper or plastic wrap, and then tighten the lid over that. Be sure to label and date. Let the kalooa steep, shaking the jar every few days. Wait at least 2 weeks before straining again as above and decanting into gift bottles. If you buy the liquor in pint bottles, those will work well.

As I have mentioned many times throughout this book, I use organic ingredients whenever possible, and I also use good booze; it just tastes better. You can experiment with additional flavoring extracts such as hazelnut or cherry. I once concocted a batch of kalooa that included cinnamon, allspice, and dried, hot chilies—get out your sombrero, it's kalooa caballero!—and it tasted great on ice with a little half-and-half. I've also made the recipe using honey instead of sugar, using a little less honey because it's sweeter than sugar and adjusting the amount of water because honey is liquid. If you decide that your kalooa is too sweet, add a little brandy to make it how you like; do not add water—this will dilute the preservative properties of the liquor and sugar. As long as you follow the basic recipe, don't be afraid to experiment with different flavorings. Since it makes several small bottles, you can flavor each one differently if you choose—just be sure to label, although a blind taste-test could be fun.

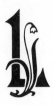 is for Lemon —
bright queen of flavors

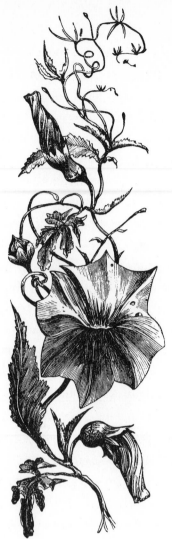

Lemons are considered to be
native to India and the Far East,
and they apparently were unknown
to the ancient Greeks and Romans.
The early Europeans learned to
cultivate lemons from the Arabs, who
had established groves well before the
Crusades of the thirteenth century.
For a time, French merchants held
a monopoly on all citrus fruits. The
Spanish established the first lemon
groves in the early 1600s in what is now
Florida. Currently, about 80 percent of the United States' crop grows
in California. While cultivated varieties do not grow true from seed,
there are at least fifteen cultivars of *Citrus limon* around the world, as
well as many other members of the Rutaceae, or rue, family, of which
the lemon is one.

Lemons Are Healthy

In terms of health and nutrition, lemons are best known for their bioflavonoid content, which helps strengthen the inner lining of the blood vessels, veins, and capillaries. The peel contains the antioxidant vitamin C and a volatile oil that is antiseptic and antibacterial, and is said to kill staph, strep, typhoid, and bacterial meningitis. (This does not mean you should eat lemon peels to cure said conditions.) The peel, in fact, is the part that contains the flavonoids; you can add some washed, chopped organic lemon, including the yellow peel and white membrane, to smoothies or salads to obtain these nutrients instead of taking a vitamin tablet. Yes, it will taste somewhat bitter, but bitters are also a digestive stimulant. As for the lemon juice, although it is acidic, once digested it has an alkaline effect and is very balancing. Lemon juice is tonic to the liver and pancreas, and you can drink plain, unsweetened lemon water for this effect; it tastes wonderful. Lemon has an antihistamine effect and reduces inflammation; I suspect lemon water may help relieve the symptoms of hay fever as well.

Perhaps some of the best-known home remedies using lemon are for coughs and colds. Hot honey-lemonade comes to mind: simply boil a cup of water, squeeze in lemon to taste, and stir in a small dab of honey. You don't have to be sick to like it, and if it's close to bedtime, you could add a dash of whisky (depending on your age) for a good night's sleep. Remember not to give honey (or whisky) to babies. Another hot lemon remedy for cold symptoms is a tea made with a pounded garlic clove, a squeeze of lemon, a pinch of cinnamon, and a dab of honey. The following lemony cold and flu combination includes health-enhancing herbs.

. . . .

Lemony Cold and Flu Tea

Boil 1 cup water; add 1 tablespoon chopped lemon peel and a pinch each sage and thyme (fresh or dried), then steep 15 minutes. Strain, then add the juice of half a lemon and a small dab of honey. Drink at least twice a day.

Lemons Are Tasty

Lemon is one of the commonest and most beloved of flavorings. From lemon cheesecake and salty Moroccan preserved lemons to icy Italian lemonade to honey-lemon roast chicken glaze (a recipe I helped my dad create for a contest—no, we didn't win), lemon is by far the brightest queen of flavors. I can't imagine a kitchen without lemons; I use them all the time. What follows are just a few of hundreds of recipes that feature lemons. As always, I recommend using organic whenever possible. I don't see how you could wash off pesticide residue anyway, as it's in the food as well as on it.

This Greek-inspired comfort food can be enjoyed hot or cold, and it makes 1 quart.

. . . .

Egg-Lemon Soup with Rice

4 cups basic chicken broth (see page 99,
  "C is for Chicken Soup")

¼ cup arborio rice (a special short-grain Italian risotto
  rice that cooks up creamy rather than grainy—use
  long-grain white rice if you can't find it)

3 egg yolks

¼ cup fresh lemon juice, strained (1–2 medium lemons)

Salt and pepper

In a medium saucepan, bring broth to boiling. Reduce heat to simmer, add the rice and a pinch of salt, then cover partially and simmer about 20 minutes until the rice is tender, stirring occasionally. Remove from heat. Meanwhile, in a mixing bowl, whisk together egg yolks and lemon juice until frothy. After rice is cooked, take 1 cup hot broth and very slowly pour it into the egg-lemon mixture, whisking constantly. Return mixture to saucepan, whisking to prevent curdling. Stir at low heat for about 5 minutes. Do not boil! Season with salt and pepper. If desired, fresh, chopped parsley makes a pretty garnish. This soup should not be reheated once chilled.

This next recipe is a classic lemony combination and is perfect for spooning over steamed veggies such as asparagus or green beans, or as a dip for artichokes.

· ·

Lemon Butter with Capers

1 cup butter (2 sticks)

2 tablespoons fresh lemon juice (about 1 lemon)

2 tablespoons capers, rinsed and patted dry

1 tablespoon minced fresh parsley, preferably flat-leaf

Melt butter slowly over low heat. Add remaining ingredients and warm through. Simple and elegant.

Although lavender isn't commonly used in the kitchen except maybe in French seasoning blends, it has a very interesting quality. Here, as a flavoring to old-fashioned lemonade, it is unbelievably refreshing. A special thanks to Jayne for introducing me to this delightful beverage.

· ·

Lavender Lemonade

1 cup water

2 tablespoons dried lavender flowers

½ cup sugar, or to taste

½ cup fresh lemon juice (2–3 lemons)—pick out the seeds

4 cups water

Boil 1 cup water, remove from heat, add lavender, stir, and then cover and steep 10 minutes. Meanwhile, combine sugar, lemon juice, and 4 cups water in a large pitcher or jar, stirring well to dissolve sugar. Strain lavender tea through a fine mesh, then add to the lemonade. Chill well, and serve over ice.

This next idea is so sweet and simple; you must try it at least once this summer. I learned about it from a Martha Stewart publication, and I can't find the original source, but you can still give her credit for it.

. . . .

Dainty Ice Cubes

Take an empty ice cube tray, fill halfway, and place a tiny lemon wedge in each cube section; freeze until mostly set, then add more water to fill the rest of the way. Freeze completely, then use with iced tea or the lemonade recipe above. Naturally, you can use a lime wedge as well, or a mint leaf, or a slice of strawberry or peach—whatever seems like a good idea at the time.

Along these same lines, you can freeze thin slices of lemon on a parchment paper-lined baking sheet. Transfer to a freezer bag, and use like an ice cube to chill and flavor a drink at the same time.

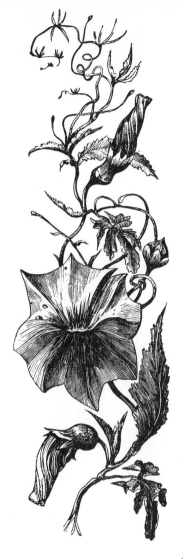

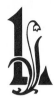

is for Lemon Balm—
sweet melissa

I may as well tell you now so I can get it over with: this herb is one of my favorite wild "domesticated" herbs, and I like all the herbs in my garden. Yes, it is available in all the garden centers, greenhouses, and seed catalogs; but let me tell you, once you have established this plant in your environs, it will likely be there for a long time, and not always where you think you planted it. Several years ago, I planted four separate lemon balm starts in an area that I no longer use as a garden. For some reason, this hardy perennial did not grow well on this site, and I thought I had lost it. Then, when the area where we garden now became more established, here was lemon balm, popping up all over the place. I couldn't believe it. I guess it wanted to be in a different spot, and now it is. It doesn't send out runners quite as wildly as its cousins spearmint or apple mint, but it does spread. And if you gently nudge it out of your garden beds and into the borders and edges here and there, you will be rewarded with a lemony fragrance that will stop you in your tracks and entice you into wanting more. Sweet Melissa, she's just that way.

How to Use Lemon Balm as a Remedy

Lemon balm (*Melissa officinalis*), also called balm and, more commonly, Melissa, is an important bee-attracting plant; in Latin, *melissa* means "bee," and this plant has been cultivated for over 2,000 years in the Mediterranean just for the bees. Medieval Arab physicians, who had a very advanced repertoire, introduced it to European herbal medicine; they used it for anxiety and depression. In fact, lemon balm is a safe, simple nervine and sedative with no negative side effects. Just take as a mild tea: boil 1 pint of water, add 2 teaspoons dried lemon balm leaf, remove from heat, and cover, steeping for 10 minutes; strain and serve. Lemon balm tea is safe for children. As a gentle anti-spasmodic, lemon balm can be taken for menstrual cramps or diarrhea. Also useful as a comforting tea for head colds and fevers, lemon balm has shown some antiviral activity, and it can be taken internally as tea and used externally as a wash for cold sores and herpes (keeping in mind that lemon balm is not a cure for these systemic viruses but a remedy for the symptoms). You can even use lemon balm in the bath and for steam facials. Rub the fresh leaf on bug bites for a quick itch-be-gone remedy.

Ways to Use Lemon Balm in the Kitchen

Lemon balm is a useful and flavorful herb with many possibilities. You don't need to be anxious to drink the tea as a beverage, and it is delicious iced. I have even made popsicles with lemon balm tea; just make it a little stronger than if you would for a beverage and sweeten to taste with sugar, since honey doesn't freeze. I include it in the fresh, chopped herbs for my spring salads. Although I have never made it myself, it is supposed to make a nice jelly. Lemon balm has been used to flavor wine and is one of the ingredients used in liqueurs such as Benedictine and Chartreuse.

Here is a recipe for a lemon balm and basil pesto with almonds, similar to one found in *The Healing Herbs Cookbook* by Pat Crocker. Try it on steamed veggies, grilled fish, or your favorite pasta.

. . . .

Lemon Balm Pesto with Almonds

2 cloves garlic

¼ cup whole almonds

2 cups fresh basil leaves, torn and packed

½ cup chopped lemon balm leaves

¼ cup grated Parmesan cheese

1 teaspoon lemon zest

¼ cup almond oil or olive oil (I think extra-
virgin is too strong for this dish)

2 tablespoons fresh lemon juice (about half a large lemon)

Salt and pepper, if desired

Mince garlic by hand or in a food processor (I have a mini processor, and I love it). Add almonds and pulse until chopped but not buttery. Next, add basil, lemon balm, cheese, and zest. Process until thoroughly chopped. Add oil and lemon juice, and process until blended to your liking. I like to add a little salt and not much pepper.

There is a curious concoction from the early seventeenth century called *Eau de Melissa Carmes,* or Carmelite Water, and it was supposedly invented by the Carmelite order of nuns (some sources say monks) in Paris in 1611. It was used as a perfume as well as a cordial, having a nervine effect as well as being useful for headaches—just imagine, drinking your perfume! Besides lemon balm, most recipes for Carmelite Water include angelica, coriander seed, nutmeg, clove, and cinnamon. Here is a recipe similar to one I found by accident (I was looking up something else) on recipezaar.com. I'm surprised I hadn't come across one sooner, since I have studied herbs for many years. I decided to add a touch of sweetener for taste.

. . . .

Carmelite Water
A Curious Cordial

>   4 tablespoons dried lemon balm leaves
>   3 tablespoons dried angelica leaves
>   2 tablespoons whole cloves
>   1 tablespoon whole coriander seed
>   1–2 teaspoons natural sugar or to taste
>   1 teaspoon freshly grated nutmeg
>   1 cinnamon stick
>   2 cups good-quality vodka

Place all the herbs, spices, and the sugar in a clean quart jar. Pour the vodka over all, adding more if necessary to cover completely. Place a small piece of waxed paper between the jar and the lid, and cover tightly; label and date. Shake every day for 3 to 4 weeks. After this time, strain the Carmelite Water into a clean decanter. This cordial will keep about six months in a cool, dark place. If you can't find angelica leaves, use 1 tablespoon dried celery leaves instead.

Do This as a Favor to Your Garden

If you grow a vegetable garden, you definitely want lemon balm around. All gardeners and orchardists know how important bees are to their crops. Some flowers require bees to assist in pollination because of their shape or location on the plant; for instance, squash blossoms are usually tucked under the leaves, so wind is not much of a help in pollination—they need bees. You can attract them by growing a pretty, lemony-smelling, lemony-tasting herb named for just them, in recognition of their value.

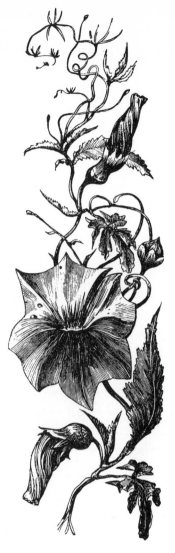

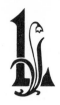

is for Lustrous
Locks —
*herbal treatments
for the hair*

Herbal concoctions can indeed add luster to your locks, and the result is shiny hair, healthy hair, truly your crowning glow-ry. What I've listed below are wild plants and garden herbs and flowers traditionally used on the hair and scalp that grow in my vicinity. Although other regions and cultures may use different plants, I like to forage locally if at all possible. I have categorized these herbs and listed them further on in the chapter.

Herbal hair treatments include those for dandruff, olde-timey growth stimulants, tonics, dyes or colorants, and homemade shampoo using castile soap. Some of the herbs fall into more than one category. There are also plants such as soapwort (*Saponaria officinalis*) and yucca (*Yucca* spp.) that contain saponins and actually make a sudsy lather in water, certainly not like your grandma's Prell or anything (thankfully), but these plants have been used for millennia for external cleansing. All the treatments discussed are for both men and women. However, if using colorants for the beard, for example, stick to the milder, less aromatic herbs, and remember that you can still shave if you make it the wrong color! If you are using herbal shampoos or hair rinses for children, dilute them to half-strength. And although these brews are made with family-friendly herbs, they are made stronger than usual, so do not drink.

Herbal Hair Tea

The simplest way to use herbs on your hair is to make a strong tea or decoction of your chosen herbs, strain into a wide bowl (with spent herbs going to the compost), and place the bowl in a deep sink or tub. Lean into the tub so that your head and hair is over the bowl, and pour cupfuls of the warm brew repeatedly over your hair until thoroughly wetted, catching what you pour back into the bowl. Continue pouring and working it into your hair and scalp until the brew is too cold for comfort. At this point, you can either rinse with lukewarm water or wrap in a dark towel (to prevent staining), then dry and style.

To make herbal hair tea, use 1 quart water to 1 or 2 handfuls of plant material (you may need more water and herbs for longer hair). This hair potion will keep in the refrigerator for about 3 days. You can also use herbal hair tea as a scalp treatment by rubbing it into your scalp every day or two, depending on what condition you are dealing with. I think you can overdo it with regular shampooing, especially in the dry cold of winter. While the scalp still needs conditioning, the hair can get dry and brittle. Most commercial shampoos are detergents that strip the hair and scalp of any natural oils and acidity it may have had; they may, in fact, overstimulate the scalp into making more oils. So the tonic treatments are a good thing, restoring the scalp and hair follicles with new vigor.

Messy but Fun

An alternative method of herbal hair treatment, and one that requires significantly more plant material, is to use dried powdered herbs and make an herbal pack for the hair and scalp. This is can be used as a dye technique. Several different herbs can be used, but the most common is the exotic henna, which is often mixed with strong, hot coffee and aromatics such as clove, nutmeg, and ginger (at least that's how I used to make it). Before you begin, tie your hair up, if possible, and run a smear of petroleum jelly or similar substance on your forehead and neck at the hairline, and the backs of your ears, just so your skin doesn't take on any stain. You'll need 4 to 8 ounces of powdered plant material to do this, depending on how long your hair is. Use boiling water—or hot coffee or tea, if you have dark hair—to make a runny paste, probably at least 1 pint, a little at a time. Add more hot water if necessary to keep it easy to work and spread; once it's cool enough—and you still want it fairly warm—apply to the hair in sections, from the scalp to the ends, then roll up each section and clip it to keep it out of the way.

Keep in mind that this will make a mess, so plan accordingly, i.e., newspapers on the floor, towels over your grubby clothes, rubber gloves, a helpful friend who has sworn not to take your picture with their cell phone, etc. Once the pack is in place, wrap your hair with plastic wrap, put a dark towel around your neck, and just sit tight for about 20 minutes. Keep the paper towels handy to wipe up any drips. Rinse thoroughly and then shampoo.

Tiny Bubbles

You can make your own specially formulated herbal shampoo—how cool is that? It's much gentler on your hair, and the cost is minimal.

. . . .

Homemade Herbal Shampoo

Take 1 pint boiling water, toss in a big handful of herbs appropriate for your hair type (see "Dyes or Colorants," page 204), reduce heat to a simmer, and steep for 20 minutes, adding more hot water to keep it at roughly 1 pint if the liquid evaporates. Line a colander with cheese-cloth, place in a bowl, and strain the brew. Remove strainer, then stir in 2 ounces grated castile soap or 2 ounces liquid castile soap to the herbal brew. Stir until the soap is melted, cool, and pour into a sham-poo bottle.

When choosing what herbs to use, try to formulate it with some-thing from each category, including a tonic, stimulant, color enhancer, and cleansing herb. You may find that a little goes a long way with this natural soap shampoo compared to most commercial brands, and you can dilute it to suit your lather requirements.

What Condition Your Conditioner Is In

Herbs steeped in vinegar is a very good final rinse for the hair after shampooing. Even plain apple cider vinegar will do. If your hair is very coarse or dry, the following conditioner can be used sparingly, after shampooing but while your hair is still wet, to give it some shine. Boil 1 pint water, add 1 large pinch each (fresh or dried) rosemary and lavender leaves, remove from heat, then cover and steep 15 minutes. Strain, then funnel into a bottle and add 2 ounces almond oil. Shake, shake, shake to disperse, then pour a small amount into your hand and gently work into your wet hair, especially the ends. Wrap in a towel until dampened off, then comb your hair with your fingers and let air dry. You might try using a spray bottle for this application, but I sus-pect it might clog up from the oil. This conditioner will keep for about 1 week.

For deep conditioning, you can give yourself a hot oil treatment. The best oils for this are avocado and almond, although you can use sunflower or jojoba oil by itself, like many of our Native American forebears did. Jojoba oil is very similar to our own skin and hair oils, and it has a long tradition in Indian and Mexican grooming as a hair restorative. Indigenous people of the Pacific Islands and coastal Asia traditionally use fragrant coconut oil on the hair, scalp, and skin. You can add a few drops of essential oil such as rosemary or lavender to the oil treatment, or you can plan ahead and make a compound oil such as for herbal salves, without the beeswax (see "The Kitchen Apothecary," beginning on page 3, for instructions on how to prepare herbal oils) and use almond oil. To prepare the hot oil hair treatment, take about 4 ounces oil (a little more if your hair is long) and heat it gently in a double-boiler fashion; I usually place the oil in a small canning jar inside a small saucepan filled with just enough water so the jar doesn't float. Slowly heat until warm, remove from the pan, and add rosemary or lavender oil if using. Dip your fingers in the oil, then rub into your scalp, a small section at a time. Once you treat the scalp, go ahead and do the strands, especially the ends. Wrap your hair in a plastic bag (it sounds worse than it is) and then an old towel. After 15 to 20 minutes, rinse as much as you can with plain warm water, then shampoo with your homemade herbal shampoo. Finish with a vinegar rinse.

Another plant used by Native Americans of the Sonora region is creosote bush (*Larrea tridentata*). This plant is also known as chapparal and has a very strong aroma. It was effectively used for dry skin, dandruff, and brittle hair. Recent research has uncovered an isolate of this plant that apparently "was found to suppress HIV-1 replication in human cells," according to a paper published by Karla Krompegel on the Colorado State University website.

Don't Flake Out

If you have dandruff, here's a recipe for a final rinse that sounds as if Simon & Garfunkle made it up: parsley, sage, rosemary, and thyme. You can also make a vinegar rinse with these herbs. The parsley is for shine, the sage is for cleansing, the rosemary is an all-around hair tonic, and the thyme is mildly medicinal. This combination is best used by those with dark hair.

Another good tonic for dandruff combines equal parts nettle leaf, violet leaf, red clover, and peppermint. Red clover contains salicylic acid, similar to aspirin, and many dandruff shampoos contain this compound; how nice it is to utilize the whole plant to include its other soothing properties.

To make these dandruff treatments, follow the method used in the "Herbal Hair Tea" section on page 198.

Toning and Stimulating

Herbal hair tonics normalize the scalp and bring it back into balance, whether overactive (oily) or dry. Some herbs can be used according to hair color. Growth stimulants are not the herbal version of Rogaine but a type of tonic that has traditionally been used (along with proper nutrition and exercise) to stimulate new hair growth. Rosemary is a good example of a hair tonic herb. Catnip is said to be an old Gypsy remedy for hair loss. A strong decoction using the inner bark of the hemlock tree (*Tsuga* spp.) is another remedy, briskly rubbed into the scalp. (Do not confuse the hemlock tree with the poisonous water hemlock, which looks like a really hurky wild carrot with purple-streaked stems. Obviously, a tree is not a carrot, but this does not go without saying.)

I might add a note to the gents here that wearing a hat all the time is not good for your scalp or hair, which needs to breathe and see the light of day; it may even contribute to hair loss.

Color Me Pretty

There are several plants, in addition to Persian, Indian, or Egyptian henna, that add subtle coloring and highlights to the hair, some for blonds, some for brunettes, and some for redheads and gray or silver (some henna formulations are neutral and do not add any color but do offer shine and strength). I wouldn't recommend using any of these plant dyes on white hair unless you're very adventurous. Use the same method of repeated rinsing as described in the section above, and be careful about splashing. You could also use the powdered herb pack method.

Categories of Use

What follows are lists of herbs according to category of best use. As mentioned, some of these will be on more than one list (this should give you a clue about the versatility of herbs and why they are so valued). Rosemary is a good place to start for dark hair; use chamomile for light hair.

Tonics

- birch leaf or twig
- horsetail (also known as scouring rush)
- juniper berries
- nettles
- rosemary
- sage leaf
- yarrow flowers

Dandruff

- apple cider vinegar
- birch bark
- hollyhock flower
- nettles
- peppermint
- red clover blossom

- rose petal
- rosemary
- sage
- violet leaf
- willow bark

Growth Stimulants

- catnip
- clove (small amount)
- hemlock tree bark
- nettles
- rosemary

Dyes or Colorants

- chamomile flower—light
- elderberries—dark (experiment on a hidden strand first, as this could turn out blue!)
- grape leaves—dark
- green walnut husks—brown (be sure to wear gloves, as this definitely stains)
- henna—store-bought, but nothing compares for warm, reddish tones
- hollyhock flowers—according to color
- marigold petals (both calendula and common garden marigolds)—light and golden
- mulberries—ditto as per elderberries, except this turns out purplish black
- mullein leaf and flower—golden
- poppy petals—red or golden

- raspberry leaves — dark

- rhubarb root — golden

- rose petals — according to color

- sage — for luster, not really a dye

- sandalwood powder (small amount) — red or golden

- St. John's wort flowering tops — red or golden

She's So Unusual

I found the following concoction referenced in more than one place, and it's so unusual that I had to include it here. And besides that, my Grandma Lil often used parsnips in her soups and stews, so it seemed right to include it. This recipe is for a hot oil pack, and the oil has to be prepared first, but it's supposed to be a marvelous hair treatment. It is my first impulse to add garlic to any simmering oil, but this is neither the time nor the place.

. . . .

Parsnip Hair Conditioner

Take 1 parsnip root, scrub clean, trim, then chop small and simmer in ¼ cup almond oil; toss in a pinch of parsnip seed if you have it. Simmer on low for 30 minutes and strain, pressing out as much oil as possible from the root. After cooling slightly, apply to scalp first and then the hair as a hot oil treatment, following the directions above.

You may find it interesting to note that many of the hair dye plants mentioned above are also used to dye wool and other fibers, and Easter eggs as well. When used with different mordants (minerals or chemicals that help the dye chemically adhere to either the protein of hair fibers or the cellulose fibers of cotton, flax, and so on), some dye plants actually make a wide range of colors. It's quite an art, and one which I have not pursued in becoming skilled at, thus far.

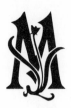

is for Mango Salsa
with Cilantro

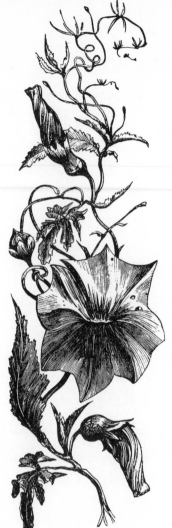

This salsa is excellent with plain boiled shrimp, scallop or shrimp kabobs, or grilled chicken. There is no reason not to replace the mangoes with fresh peaches, nectarines, or plums if they are ripe and beckoning, which is the wild and weedy way.

Enjoy mango salsa during the height of summer's bounty, when the herbs, fruits, and veggies will be at their peak. If you have a baby around, you can give them the sweet, pulpy mango pit to chew on, which is quite large and difficult for them to get their mouth around.

· ·

Mango Salsa with Cilantro

2 mangoes, fully ripe, coarsely chopped (about 3 cups)

1 jalapeño pepper, minced (remove ribs
   and seeds if you like it mild)

1 red bell pepper, chopped

1 small red onion, finely chopped

3 scallions, white part with a bit of green, sliced

¼ cup chopped cilantro

Juice of 1 lime

Juice of 1 sweet orange

Cayenne pepper, optional

Cut mangoes in half and remove pit. If you've never cut open a mango before, the pit is large and long and flat, and you basically cut around the pit. Scoop pulp out from skin (discard skin) and chop. (If you are using peaches, peel them; plums and nectarines are fine with the skins on.) Combine all ingredients and refrigerate at least 30 minutes. Then taste for heat and add cayenne if deemed necessary. This salsa is pretty mild in spite of the onion and jalapeño.

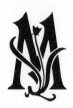

is for Mint—
very refreshing

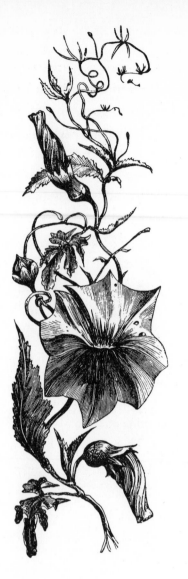

I hardly know where to start.
Here are some of the more popular
and easy-to-locate members of the
mint family:

- apple mint
- chocolate mint
- Corsican mint
- ginger mint
- grapefruit mint
- lemon mint
- lime mint
- orange mint, also known as bergamot
  mint and eau de cologne mint
- pennyroyal
- peppermint
- pineapple mint
- spearmint
- wild mint, or field mint

As you can see, there is a wide variety of mint, some with sub-varieties of their own. For instance, amongst the spearmint group, there is curly mint, Scotch mint, English mint, and Kentucky Colonel mint (bringing to mind mint juleps) — as well as others. Chocolate mint is a type of peppermint with a distinctive "peppermint patty" aroma. Corsican mint is a low-growing ground cover with delicate, rounded leaves and does well in the rock garden. Orange mint is luscious and beautiful; the name bergamot is the same as another mint relative called bergamot or, more properly, monarda (neither of which is related to the bergamot orange, wherefrom the essential oil is derived). Field mint is decidedly musky, with a strong menthol flavor and aroma. Most mints do not breed true from seed and must be propagated by cuttings. Spearmint is an important trade crop in the state of Washington, where I have seen vast fields of the herb, lush and green and pulsating with energy.

Once you grow one or two varieties of mint, you will likely want to grow others; just don't grow the different types in the same bed or next to each other or they will probably cross-pollinate and lose their individuality. Mint is a good container plant, and one way to make a permanent container is to plant it in a terra-cotta chimney flue; they're usually about two feet long, so you can sink it at least a foot into the ground and then do your planting within the flue. It still might send runners down and around the barrier, though; as I mentioned, mint is quite energetic.

Mint in the Kitchen

While most of us have had a cup of peppermint tea purely for pleasure, many of the mints are useful as a culinary herb. Spearmint combines nicely with cucumbers, and is used, in combination with parsley, in the Middle Eastern salad called tabbouleh. It's also combined with dill and fresh salmon in the Scandinavian preparation gravlax (see page 119). Here is a recipe for a mint-infused wine inspired by one found in *The Herbal Pantry* by Emelie Tolley and Chris Mead. Naturally, I tweaked it a bit to appease my own personal preferences, which is what I encourage you to do as well. It's a delightful refreshment for a summer picnic.

. . . .

White Wine with Orange and Mint

¼ **cup water**

¼ **cup sugar**

¼ **cup orange mint or spearmint**

3 strips orange zest

1 bottle (1 fifth) dry white wine

¼ **cup brandy**

2 tablespoons orange flower water (find this at imported foods or Middle Eastern groceries)

Combine the water and sugar in a small saucepan and heat until the sugar is thoroughly dissolved, then cool to lukewarm. Place the mint and orange zest in a quart-sized glass jar, then pour the sugar syrup over and stir. Let cool. Next, add the wine, brandy, and orange flower water. Place a piece of waxed paper on top of the jar, then close the lid over that. Steep in a cool, dark place for 2 or 3 days, and then filter into an appropriate decanter. Chill before serving. Garnish with fresh mint if desired.

You might want to try fixing apple mint relish (found on page 53) using either the spearmint or pineapple mint—or both. I have recently discovered a whole carnival of specialty (trademarked) mints from Richter's herb, seed, and plant company from Ontario, Canada; many unusual, fruit-scented *Mentha* varieties such as Berries & Cream and Sweet Pear await the adventurous mint enthusiast. Richter's has been around for a decades, and it's doubtful they'll go away anytime soon.

Home Remedies Using Mint

Peppermint is a local anesthetic to the nerves of the stomach and intestinal tract. You can have a cup of tea before eating to increase bile production, which is important for proper digestion. Peppermint tea is reputedly safe to drink for morning sickness during pregnancy, as it does not stimulate the uterus—but ask your midwife just to be sure, and never use peppermint essential oil during pregnancy. You can combine peppermint with yarrow and elderflower as a tea to relieve flu symptoms accompanied by fever: boil 1 pint water and add 1 teaspoon each dried mint leaf, yarrow flower and elderflower; remove from heat and steep for 10 minutes, then strain and serve. While peppermint tea is very effective for relieving nausea and stomach or menstrual cramps, spearmint is more appropriate for children's complaints, including headache, plus they love the flavor and aroma—and who doesn't? I always keep around a tin or two of those curiously strong peppermints known as Altoids for instant nausea relief and have been amazed at their effectiveness.

Externally, the mints make a soothing and refreshing bath herb that is of benefit to rashes such as chicken pox, while the analgesic properties help soothe a sore, achy body. Mint combines nicely with seaweed in the bath—see "B is for Bathing Beautiful," page 70, for how to prepare herbs for the bath. Used in a steam facial, mint is cleansing and stimulating; just boil up a bit of water in a small saucepan, throw in a couple pinches of mint leaf, stir, then sit at the table with your face over the pan and a towel over your head, steaming for about 10 minutes. I include fresh mint when making grandma's magic healing salve (see page 147); just like garden thyme, mint also contains the antiseptic thymol.

It's Greek to Me

Mint is native to the Near East and Mediterranean regions. During biblical times, it was used as a tithe and a medium of exchange.

Says Mrs. M. Grieve in *A Modern Herbal*, "in Athens, where every part of the body was perfumed with a different scent, mint was specially designated to the arms." The aroma of mint, even the fruity varieties, tends to animate or energize the spirit, bringing a feeling of brightness and clarity. Mint was often used as a strewing herb for this reason, especially during illness. While most of us don't strew herbs around the house these days, fresh mint in vases or even bundled and hung to dry lend an atmosphere of cheer and optimism.

Since it has been overcast all day and kind of dreary outside, I think a cup of peppermint tea would be perfect right about now to refresh my computer-screen brainspace.

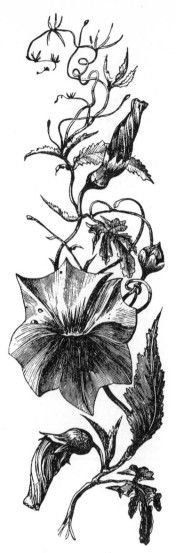

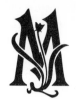

is for Morel
Mushroom Gratin

This rich gratin is best prepared
with the wild morel mushroom, but
you can use button mushrooms if
the morels are unavailable. For me,
morel mushrooms cause a dewy-eyed,
nostalgic remembering of previous
years' great noshes. Rarely available
domestically, their season is short-
lived and highly anticipated. The fresh
herbs in the recipe ought to be available
in the garden at the same time the
mushrooms are popping up in the field.

. . . .

Morel Mushroom Gratin

1 pound fresh morel mushrooms, stems removed

1 tablespoon olive oil

2 tablespoons butter

½ cup cream

1½ cups fresh bread crumbs

1 tablespoon snipped fresh chives

2 teaspoons fresh thyme leaves

4 tablespoons butter, melted

Preheat oven to 375 degrees. Slice the mushrooms into rings. Heat olive oil in a large, heavy skillet to medium hot, and then add 2 tablespoons butter. Add mushrooms and briefly sauté, then pour into a 9-inch glass pie pan. Pour cream over the mushrooms. Toss together bread crumbs, chives, thyme, and the melted butter in a bowl, and sprinkle evenly over the mushrooms and cream, lightly pressing down to even the surface. Bake for 25–30 minutes or until crisp and golden.

This is *so-o-o-o* good!

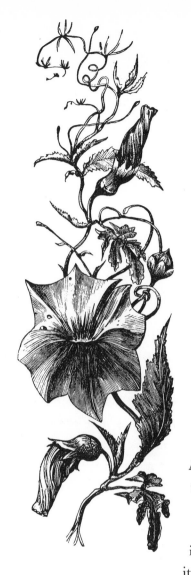

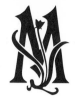

is for Mother's
Tummy Rub

This is a delightful and deliciously
fragrant balm for rubbing on the
expanding abdomen of the mother-
to-be, and for after the birthing as
well. It even makes a tasty lip balm.
After you have gathered and dried
the botanicals from your garden,
it doesn't take long to make. You
might want to get your older children
in on the action, including rubbing
it on your belly. The simple, loving
gesture of helping care for The Mama
will in turn nurture the growing babe-in-waiting. I have many times
witnessed young children talking to their mother's bellies—the baby
inside, that is—and it really doesn't get any cuter. It can be a time to
prepare the older children for the changes to come, especially if they
are only children without siblings; not being Number One anymore
can bring out the spoiled brat in any kid (including the daddy-to-be).
This balm can be a soothing interface for the necessary adjustments of

cooperative family life. Cocoa butter is a well-known component used to prevent stretch marks. I have a friend who has had six children, and her belly is smooth as can be, thanks to Mother's Tummy Rub, along with plenty of good food, fresh air, and walking. Purchase cocoa butter at a pharmacy, health food store, or your favorite confectionary supply. This balm smells good enough to eat, and basically, it is edible.

· ·

Mother's Tummy Rub

    1 cup almond oil

    ½ cup dried calendula flower petals

    ½ cup dried rose petals

    1 ounce grated beeswax

    ½ ounce cocoa butter, cut into small pieces

    1 teaspoon vitamin E oil (or just squeeze 2
        vitamin E capsules into the mix)

Steep the oil and dried flower petals over very low heat for at least 2 hours; if you have a mini slow cooker, use that, and let steep overnight for approximately 10 hours uncovered. If warming on a stove top, turn off heat overnight and cover with a towel; continue warming the next day for about 8 hours. Don't worry about precise timing, just don't let the flower petals burn. Strain out the botanicals. Next, stir the beeswax and cocoa butter into the warm oil until melted, then add the vitamin E oil. Pour into convenient wide-mouth containers (2 half-pint canning jars work especially well), and if there's any leftover, pour into tiny lip-balm pots.

I would recommend taking loads of photos during this magical time, as each pregnancy is unique. As your children grow, you will all share in the memories, especially when they're old enough to start dating and you take out their baby pictures.

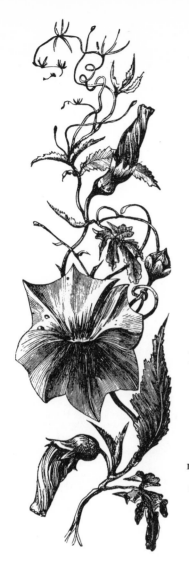

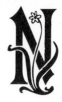

is for Nacho Pie

Yes, the title of this recipe sounds
like something that would have been
served to the Brady Bunch, but it is
so easy and cheesy that I think it is
a boon to the repertoire of any busy
kitchen-witchy mom with hordes
massing at the screen door. You can
defend yourself with carrot sticks and
douse them with lemonade while the
pie is in the oven.

. . . .

Nacho Pie

2 eggs, beaten

2 cups crushed tortilla chips (approximately 6–8 ounces)

**2 cups (6–8 ounces) grated jack cheese,
  or your favorite combination**

1 (12-ounce) jar chunky salsa

1 (4-ounce) can green chilies, rinsed and sliced into strips

Chopped fresh cilantro

Sour cream, optional

Heat oven to 400 degrees. Grease a 12-inch glass pie pan or other wide, shallow casserole. Combine eggs and crushed chips in a large bowl, mixing well. Press mixture evenly onto bottom and sides of prepared pan. Bake 10 minutes, then remove from oven. Sprinkle on most of the cheese, then the cilantro, some or all of the salsa, and arrange the chilies, then top with the remaining cheese. Bake until cheese is melted, about 10 minutes. Let rest a couple minutes, and then cut into wedges to serve. Top with sour cream, if desired.

The green chilies and cilantro are just some of many options that can go into the pie; other examples include sliced olives, chopped onions or scallions, cooked beans, or even a little leftover cooked meat. If you don't have salsa, use fresh sliced tomatoes and minced peppers. I like lots of greens and veggies with all that cheese; use what you like best. I have found that grated carrot can find its way into a lot of places (such as the crust; about 2 grated carrots should do).

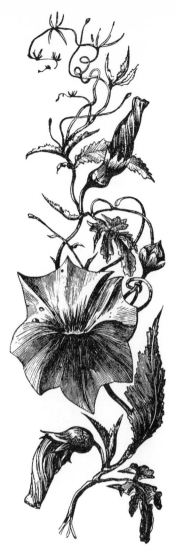

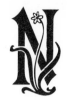

is for Nettles—
don't be afraid!

People usually recoil at the sight
or even mention of stinging nettles,
but once you learn more about
them, you'll realize they have much
nourishment to offer.

Urtica dioica is native to Europe
and naturalized in North America. It
has been suggested that nettles were
cultivated in Mexico as long as eight
thousand years ago. One of the earli-
est domestic uses of the nettle plant was
as cloth, made from the fibrous stems. In
Denmark, this nettle cloth was found in a Bronze Age burial site, probably two thousand years old. Nettle cloth is well known in Scotland,
where some say it is more fine and durable than flax. Nettle fiber is
fifty times stronger than cotton and almost as strong as silk. Cordage
made from nettle fiber is excellent, and it is a traditional fiber used for
making bowstrings, along with the closely related and equally traditional hemp fiber, which is even more durable. The very name "nettles"

comes from the German *nat-ilo* and Old English *netele*, indicating "a net" and "to tie or bind."

When picking nettles, be sure to wear gloves; both drying and cooking eliminate the sting, which is similar to an ant bite. I usually collect them bare-handed (my husband would say "people-handed"), even though I end up with a few welts that last several hours; I consider it a challenge to nip off the stems with my thumbnail and forefinger, and the numbing tingle is somewhat intriguing. Pick in early spring before they flower and become too fibrous and no longer edible. Nettles are most often found in semi-shaded, moist areas, with buttercups and violets as common companion plants; it almost resembles a large mint plant, but the flowers are quite different and so is the aroma. Please consult one of the field guides listed in the bibliography for a complete description, and do not hesitate to ask one of the old-timers in your neighborhood to show you where a good stand of nettles can be located.

In the garden area, nettles enrich the soil and can be added to the compost pile to help accelerate the process. On the farm, dried nettles can be added to chicken scratch or larger animals' fodder for greater assimilation of nutrients. In the wild, nettles indicate damp, fertile soil; you can even smell the vitality.

In the kitchen, nettles are tasty and nutritious, being a good source of calcium, iron, magnesium, potassium, silica, B vitamins (including folic acid), carotenes, a fair amount of protein for a leafy plant (7 percent), and chlorophyll. As a delicious beverage tea, they are somewhat diuretic, but they supply more minerals than they deplete. Actually, eating them is a better way to access their nutrients, especially with a glug of herbal vinegar as a dressing (which helps make the minerals more available). Cook fresh nettle leaf just like spinach, collards, or what have you—they taste a lot like the wild green earth, full of richness and vibrant energy. And when you do cook them (just the leaves or the very young tops), save the juice—and use it as a hair tonic! It helps eliminate dandruff and promotes a healthy scalp. Simply pour over the head after shampooing, massage gently into the scalp, and do not rinse. This will bring luster to the hair, especially dark or graying hair.

One way to use the already cooked and drained nettles is to find your favorite recipe for handmade pasta and replace the spinach in the fettuccini with nettles, or use the recipe for nettle noodles found in *How to Prepare Common Wild Foods* by another Idaho author and herbalist, Darcy Williamson. Boiled in salted water until al dente, then tossed with some garlic-enriched olive oil, toasted pine nuts, and a bit of grated Parmesan cheese ... need I say more?

I discovered another excellent way to use nettles from Susun Weed in her book *Healing Wise* — a flavorful seasoning that is easy to prepare.

. . . .

Sesame-Nettle Sprinkle

Toast 1 cup white sesame seeds in a heavy pan over medium heat, stirring constantly to prevent scorching, until slightly browned. Remove seeds from pan to a plate where they can cool, and then crush the seeds with a mortar and pestle or pulse them in the blender (until crumbly but not pasty) with a teaspoon of salt and ¼ cup dried, crushed nettle leaf. Used as a table condiment just like salt, but certainly more nutritious, it is similar to the Japanese gomasio, which is simply salt added to the toasted sesame seeds.

I like to throw a small handful of dried nettles into a simmering soup pot (see page 99, "C is for Chicken Soup"); in fact, this is a good way to use the dried stems since they'll be strained out anyway. It's not unusual for me to take this broth and use it to make polenta or risotto.

This final idea is one I've been using for years. Pick the nettles at their peak (which is usually mid- to late spring), dry them in bunches, strip the leaves from the stems, and use as you would dried parsley (and, as mentioned above, save the stems for broth). And when your husband or any of the other kids ask what all that green stuff is in the mashed potatoes, just smile and say, "It's herbal seasoning"... because it is.

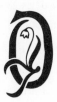

is for Oats

Feelin' yours lately? People have been eating and using oats for eons. Made into gruel, it can be used to gently strengthen and soothe the body during illness. Tea made from oatstraw, gathered when the heads of the grain are still in the milky stage, is used as a gentle sedative and nervine, free from side effects. I make a nerve tonic tincture out of equal parts oatstraw, lemon balm, and skullcap; over time, this combination helps bring a gradual sense of calm and balance and is not directly sedative (the recipe for making this tincture can be found in the chapter "O is for Oh, My Achin' Head!" on page 225). Oats are good food for pregnant women because of its bone-building minerals—phosphorus, magnesium, and calcium—and they also contain potassium, tocopherol, gluten, protein, and starch. Oats also are a good source of soluble fiber.

Externally, an oatmeal poultice can be used on inflammations and insect bites; just soak about 1 tablespoon of uncooked rolled oats (quick oats are quicker) in ¼ cup boiling hot water until softened and cooled a bit, then apply this paste/poultice to the site. A muslin bag of rolled oats in the bath is soothing and cleansing, and can be used to ease the discomfort of chicken pox, eczema, and so on. This is especially useful in the children's bath with the addition of calendula petals and lemon balm leaves added to the muslin bag—don't be surprised if the kid falls asleep as soon as they're out of the tub. There are many suggestions for herbal baths in "B is for Bathing Beautiful," beginning on page 70.

Oatmeal can be used as a facial cleanser. Simply grind a small amount of rolled oats in your blender, make a little paste of it with a bit of warm water in the palm of your hand (it's okay if it's still a little grainy), and wash away—don't forget your neck, you'll be amazed by the results. You can also add some ground almonds and honey to the blend, or even a little yogurt, although the temptation to try and lick it off your own face may be strong. I should mention that this procedure can be a little messy, so you might want to do this in the shower. It's okay to grind some extra oats to last a few days, just store them in a little container.

The following recipe is one of my favorite ways to use oats. It may not be what you'd call low-fat, but it is good energy food. Similar to tea snacks served in Scotland, these bannocks are comforting, fragrant biscuitlike wedges, welcome anytime but especially during cool autumn days, on long hikes, or in huntin' camp. I love them.

. . . .

Oatmeal-Cheese Bannocks

2 cups rolled oats, ground in the blender to make some fine, some coarse, plus a little extra for kneading

¼ teaspoon salt

4 tablespoons cold butter (half a stick)

1 cup (about 4 ounces) grated sharp Cheddar

½ cup warm water

Heat oven to 350 degrees, and lightly grease a baking sheet. Stir the ground oatmeal and salt together in a bowl. Grate the butter into the oatmeal, stir it up a bit, and then stir in the grated cheese. Add water a little at a time and mix, kneading by hand when dough is too stiff to stir. Divide into two parts, and then roll each part into a circle about ¼- to ½-inch thick. I find it helpful to roll out the dough between two sheets of oat-dusted waxed paper. Place on prepared baking sheet and carefully cut each circle into six wedges, or farls. Bake 20 minutes or until lightly golden. While they are delightful warm from the oven, the Cheddar flavor is stronger once they're cooled.

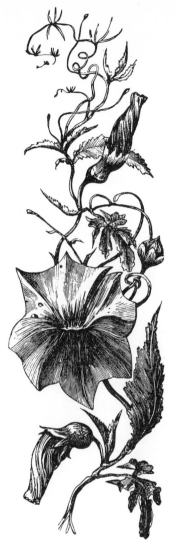

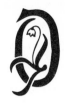

is for Oh,
My Achin' Head—
*herbal simples & other
remedies to relieve
symptoms*

My purpose here is to examine
the types and causes of headaches
and to review some of the domestic
and wild plants that can be used to
relieve the symptoms of this modern
and all-too-common ailment.

Obviously, a headache is any pain
in the head, but aside from this glib bit
of sarcasm, there may be several types of
headache, and the areas where the pain is experienced may be clues as
to the cause of the pain; traditional Chinese medicine is greatly noted
for its extensive diagnostic repertoire. For some headaches, the cause
may be obvious, such as eyestrain or lack of exercise, but some causes
may be more subtle, such as fluorescent lighting or hidden allergies.
There are easy ways to remedy most headaches once you know the
cause. Migraine headaches are much more severe, debilitating in fact,

and will not be discussed in this chapter, nor will I discuss allergy headaches. As for headaches caused by a hangover, prevention is without a doubt the best medicine.

Digestion and Headache

Most of the herbs used to facilitate digestion are also good for headaches, since indigestion can often be the precursor to a headache. A mild tea of store-bought Asian ginger root or even wild ginger root is a tasty and effective remedy. Even a good natural ginger ale can help. The fragrant wild ginger, with its low-growing, kidney-shaped leaves and unusual flower, is easy to identify and can often be found in the middle of winter since it stays ever green and prefers moist, shaded areas where snow might not accumulate so densely. To make tea from this or any type of ginger, boil 1 pint water, add 1 rounded teaspoon fresh or ½ teaspoon dried ginger root (not powder), and let steep 10 minutes. Strain and serve. If you only have ginger root powder, just put a pinch or two to a mug of boiling water and stir; it's that easy. Sweeten with a dab of honey if desired.

All the mints are good for headache and indigestion, and a tea combination of mint and alfalfa is exceptional in taste and effectiveness. Alfalfa is highly nutritious and contains digestive enzymes. Spearmint is milder than peppermint and so is a good remedy for children; so is a mild catnip tea, which also has a calming effect.

Get a Move On

Sometimes we become couch potatoes, don't get out for walks often enough, and are lazy for a spell. Our circulation becomes sluggish, and we may come to experience a dull headache. Exercise or vigorous activity can help remedy this. We can drink mint tea for its gentle stimulating effect. We can also drink hawthorn berry tea, which is a super tonic to the heart and arteries (the tincture in particular). Hawthorn berries are adaptogenic, which means that they are harmless in the absence of stress but balancing in the face of injury or stress. They are very mildly sedative. They also taste good, and I can pick them in the wild. To learn more about hawthorn berries, see "H is for Hawthorn" on page 156.

I might add here that a diet of whole grains and fresh veggies (including fresh garlic) and regular physical activity will also contribute to healthy circulation. Also, drink plenty of water to keep your body and all its organs well hydrated.

Nervous Tension

Probably the single greatest cause of headaches is nervous tension. This is going to take some lifestyle change, especially some sort of meditation technique or quiet self-nurturing. I can't *stress* this enough to the busy-to-the-point-of-frazzled moms I know: nobody can give you this time; you have to take it for yourself. And it's not selfish; think of it as a survival mechanism for modern times. The world really is moving faster than when you were a kid, and if you don't step off the merry-go-round on a regular basis, you'll wind yourself up so tight that, like a violin string, you will finally break. Don't let yourself get to that point. There are many ways to meditate and a multitude of books, audio materials, classes, and other resources to teach you how, and everybody has ten or fifteen minutes at some point in their day to take care of themselves. Lock yourself in the bathroom if you have to!

If stress is not a chronic problem for you, and you just need to zone after a busy day, herbal teas such as chamomile, catnip, lavender, lemon balm, mullein, and sage are all good for their calming effect. Just the act of preparing a pot of tea has the quality of slowing one down, and taking the time to crush and smell the herbs and to quietly care for yourself or a loved one is without a doubt very effective in calming the nerves. As you inhale the steaming aroma and sip the fragrant brew, you can visualize the tea soothing away the tension that caused your headache. Feel your nerves relax, and release all attachment to the troubles at hand, knowing that nothing can be solved through anxiety.

Here is a recipe for an herbal tincture that is not sedative but rather tonic to the nervous system, gently nourishing and calming. Follow the directions on page 10 in "The Kitchen Apothecary" for how to make tinctures.

. . . .

Nerve Tonic Tincture

Dried green oat straw

Dried skullcap herb

Dried lemon balm herb

Use equal amounts of each herb and place in a suitable jar for tincturing, keeping in mind that the dried herbs will expand somewhat (we're probably looking at ½ cup of each herb in a 1-quart jar). Use 100-proof vodka to cover, and let steep for about 2 weeks, shaking daily. Strain when ready. The usual dose for adults is 15 to 30 drops (not droppers full) when needed, 2 or 3 times a day.

A steaming brew of violet leaf tea, which contains methyl salicylate (a component of aspirin), or a cool tea of lemon balm or garden thyme are effective headache remedies. Rosemary tea, which is a gentle stimulant, is very good for headaches; I have used it quite successfully. A simple herb tea is made with 1 pint boiling water, removed from heat and steeped with 1 rounded teaspoon chosen herb for 10 minutes, then strained and served. Rosemary essential oil dabbed on the temples is another method to remedy a headache, or you could place a few drops on a cotton ball and tie it into a handkerchief and inhale the aroma. Another way to use rosemary for headaches is to make a simmering potpourri of the leaves and inhale the vapor. Do not use rosemary or any other essential oil to make tea, or during pregnancy.

Did She Really Say That?

If you've ever told your sweetie "not tonight, I have a headache," well, all I can say is shame on you. Sex is probably the most pleasurable remedy I can think of for relieving a headache or poor circulation.

And before you go looking for love in all the wrong places, don't over-
look the possibility of, ahem, dancing with yourself, as it were.

Speaking of Touch...

Therapeutic massage is also useful for relieving tension, and a quiet,
uninterrupted herb-infused bath, complete with candles, can also be a
wonderful way to relax (see "B is for Bathing Beautiful," page 70, for
more ideas on this). Fragrant, relaxing herbs such as lavender, rose
petals, lemon balm, birch leaf or bark, comfrey root or leaf, calendula,
or chamomile—the last two of which are especially good for children
—are all worthy of mention.

Other ways to use herbs for relieving headache are to crush the
leaves of yarrow and inhale the aroma, like the Shoshone Indians did,
or make a compress of pine-needle tea and lay this across the forehead. Many Native Americans have smoked the leaves of kinnikinnick, also known as bearberry or uva ursi, but rather than suggest that
you smoke anything except salmon (just the thought of it makes me
feel better), you could use the kinnikinnick as an incense or smudge
for energetic pain relief. To make a compress of these herbs, boil 1 pint
of water with a handful of pine needles, turn down to a simmer, cover,
and let steep for 10 minutes; strain and dip a soft cloth into the slightly
cooled brew and lay this to the forehead as often as necessary. Do not
drink this brew.

The crushed leaves of any fresh mint can be laid on the forehead
to relieve a headache; the leaves are somewhat analgesic and can be
made into a compress (see above) for any number of aches and pains,
particularly rheumatism. Inhaling the vapors of steeping mint tea is
helpful in relieving a sinus headache.

Other Causes of Headache—with Simple Remedies

Fluorescent lighting is known to cause headaches and other neu-
rological disorders as well. I go on sensory overload any time I walk
into a mega-mart store such as Wally World (you know the one I

mean). If you have these kinds of fixtures in your home, the tubes can be replaced with the full-spectrum variety, although you might still get that strobe effect. The newer halogen light fixtures also give off a bright light without the jarring brightness or hum of the fluorescents, so you may want to consider this option. I have found that the energy-efficient compact fluorescent bulbs give off less light than incandescent and cause me more eyestrain — what's a good dog to do? As mentioned above, excessive eyestrain can cause severe headaches. Pay special attention to your children if they complain of headaches; they may need an eye exam. It's also a good idea to limit their exposure to computer screens and video games.

Low blood sugar is another common cause of headaches, especially in children. What child doesn't come home from school hungry? A healthy snack of quality protein plus complex carbohydrates, such as cheese or meat with whole grain crackers or yogurt with fresh fruit, will help balance them, as will many other tasty combinations.

Air pollution causes headaches — amongst many other ills — and, short of relocating house and home, we can't always alleviate the cause. So rather than having a bad attitude, which will only make the pain worse ...

Go to Your Quiet Place

...your herb garden, a secluded spot in the woods, or even the privacy of your own bedroom. Just take the time to be alone, to meditate, to sing, to pray, something ... whatever works for you. Try to spend a little time each day in this contemplative frame of mind, to sip your tea and reflect on the beauty that is, and give thanks for that beauty. Give thanks for your ability to preserve and create more beauty. Relieving daily stress in this way is a sure preventative for avoiding tension headaches, and probably other illnesses as well.

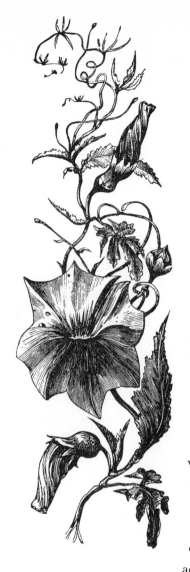

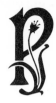 is for Parsley

Parsley is believed to have originated in Turkey and the Middle East, where it can still be found in the wild. The ancient Greeks used wreaths of parsley to adorn the tombs of the dead; they also used it to decorate the victors of the Isthmian Games, similar to our modern Olympics. Frequent consumption of parsley was said to make the nerves strong. The essential oil is sometimes used in perfumery to add a warm note.

As an herbal home remedy, a dose of simple parsley tea—1 rounded teaspoon dried leaf to 1 pint boiling water, steeped for 10 minutes—has a diuretic action; in my experience, parsley tea helps to normalize overly acidic conditions of the urinary tract. Do not use parsley tea if you are pregnant. Parsley is also very nutritious, most notably rich in beta-carotene. Parsley leaf mashed into a paste can be applied to insect stings and bites; this is called a poultice.

I highly recommend you use fresh parsley in your cooking, or dry your own. It takes a while for the seeds to germinate, but it's easy to grow. Alternatively, you could find some at the farmer's market and get a few bunches to dry at home; first, wash in cold water by grasping the stems and swishing the leaves in the water, then dry thoroughly on a towel and hang in loose bunches (secured by a rubber band) in an airy, shaded spot. I prefer the Italian flat-leaf type of parsley.

The following recipe is a refreshing way to use fresh parsley; along with cooling mint, my own version of the Middle Eastern classic tabbouleh makes an easy supper or side dish. With fresh, nutritious herbs and veggies, it's a wonderful summer salad. Paula Wolfert's *The Cooking of the Eastern Mediterranean* is an excellent reference for those interested in the authentic cooking of this ancient cultural region; it's like an armchair tour into the kitchens of the somewhere familiar yet nearly forgotten. Bulgur is a cracked, par-cooked wheat kernel that serves up quickly. Do not substitute with plain cracked wheat.

. . . .

Tabbouleh

½ cup bulgur wheat

1½ cups boiling water

2 cups chopped, fresh parsley leaves

½ cup chopped, fresh mint leaves (I use spearmint)

2 cloves chopped, fresh garlic

½ cup thinly sliced scallions (save a bit for garnish)

2 seeded and chopped tomatoes

¼ cup olive oil

½ cup fresh lemon juice (about 2 medium lemons)

Salt and pepper

6 large lettuce leaves (to use as serving cups)

In a heat-resistant bowl, soak the bulgur in boiling water for 30 minutes, until tender; it will remain chewy. In a large bowl, toss chopped herbs, garlic, and scallions with the tomato. Drain bulgar well, and add to the veggies. Pour oil and lemon over all, and add seasonings to taste. Mix well, divide equally amongst the 6 lettuce leaf cups, then garnish. Chopped cucumber makes a nice addition to this salad.

Makes 6 salads.

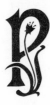 is for Plantain—
no, we are not bananas!

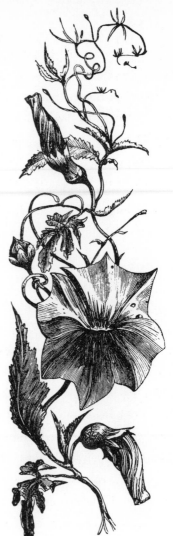

Plantain is a widespread plant no bigger than your foot that grows all over the world, from cities to mountains, and is used from Europe to Africa to Asia to the Americas. It is not the same as plantains (with an "s"), the tropical fruit that looks like a red banana on the outside and is starchy rather than sweet, plus it needs to be cooked. Our subject here is a common garden weed: the common plantain (*Plantago major*) and narrow, or lanceleaf, plantain (*P. lanceolata*) are low-growing, leafy rosettes with a circular cluster of leaves; they send up odd-looking flower spikes that some find akin to miniature cattails. One distinctive feature of plantain leaves is that all the veins run parallel lengthwise, from the leaf stem to the leaf tip. Plantain is sometimes called ribwort. Many people try to eradicate it from their lawns, but I'm a mountain gal, and if it ain't got thorns, it can stay! Besides, plantain is so useful and gregarious, I'd like everyone to know about it.

Plantain is instant first aid. Native to Europe, folklore has it that many American Indians called the common or broadleaf plantain "white man's footprint," because it grew wherever the newcomers journeyed. The Indians wasted no time, however, using plantain for all the same things the Europeans did, which is for the external treatment of just about any skin irritation or inflammation that may be encountered. Plantain, both kinds, is used for insect bites and stings, bruises, swelling from sprains, and any type of minor scrape or wound. Simply crush the fresh leaf by mashing in a mortar and pestle and apply to all manner of common irritations. If necessary, you can simply chew up the leaf in your mouth and plaster it on the sting or bite just like that (don't say *eeooouw*—it really works!). You can also make a compress for larger areas such as for sunburn or nettle rash with a cool, strong tea of the herb; dip a large, soft cloth into the tea and lay it over the affected area. Plantain helps stop bleeding, stimulates healing, is antimicrobial, and the lanceleaf variety in particular is anti-inflammatory. It has a cooling, moistening, yet drawing quality that makes any boo-boo feel better.

Plantain can also be used internally. It is the same genus as psyllium, and its leaf and seed also have mucilaginous properties. It has been used for urinary tract disorders, toning the digestive system in general, the bladder specifically, is slightly laxative, and is soothing to all mucous membranes. Plantain can be taken as a mild tea for dry or hacking respiratory conditions; take 1 rounded teaspoon dried leaf and steep in 1 pint boiling water for 10 minutes, strain, and serve.

In the olden days, plantain was used as a potherb like spinach, the young, tender leaves being the most choice.

Plantain is a very useful herb for making soothing salves, but you must make an oil extract with it first. Take one large handful fresh plantain leaves, wash and dry, then place in a medium saucepan or mini slow cooker, and cover with two cups olive oil (or more, if necessary, to cover). Set the pan, uncovered, to the lowest simmer (or turn the slow cooker to high, also uncovered) to extract the green goodness from the plantain leaf. Simmer in saucepan about 8 hours or overnight in the mini crock. Let cool, and proceed from there to make a salve (see page 13 in "The Kitchen Apothecary"), or use the plantain oil by itself as a softening massage oil for tired, hard-workin' feet.

Not until after many years of studying herbs on my part did I learn that my grandmother knew about plantain. She mostly tried to pull it out of her yard, but she did tell me once that her parents used this weed for bites, scrapes, and bruises. I was surprised at Gramma but more so at myself for never thinking to ask her about healing plants until then. I know that everyone used to eat spring dandelion greens, but I have since learned that each person is a potential font of information concerning wild plants and herbs and Grandma's home remedies. I hope I can always take the time to seek this information, try it out on myself, and pass on what works to the younger ones, who very much need a tradition they can count on.

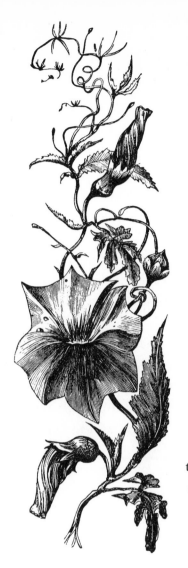

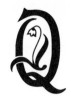

is for Q Sauce —
oh, yeah!

Who doesn't like a sweet, spicy, sticky, righteous 'que? This sauce is easy to make and is excellent on chicken or ribs, or you can use it to simmer leftover roasted and thinly sliced meat of any type for sandwiches.

· ·

Q Sauce

1 small onion, chopped

1 clove garlic, minced

1 tablespoon oil

1 (14-ounce) bottle ketchup (1¾ cup)

¼ cup molasses

2 tablespoons honey or brown sugar

1 tablespoon Tabasco sauce

1 teaspoon Worcestershire sauce

1–2 teaspoons cayenne powder, to taste

1 teaspoon prepared mustard, preferably brown

1 teaspoon chili powder

¼ teaspoon powdered ginger

In a medium saucepan over medium heat, sauté the onion in oil until tender, about 15 minutes; then add garlic until it becomes fragrant, which will be almost immediately (you don't want it to burn). Add ketchup, molasses, honey, Tabasco, Worcestershire, cayenne, mustard, chili powder, and ginger, stirring or whisking until well incorporated. Bring back to boiling, then set to a very low simmer for 20 minutes, stirring occasionally.

After simmering the sauce, if you will be swabbing grilled meat, do so according to your own personal tradition—you must have experience with outdoor grilling—and be sure to wait until the meat is mostly done to baste with this sauce; otherwise, it will burn. Alternatively, use it as an afterburner or dipping sauce.

If you are making sandwiches with leftover sliced meat, add the meat to the sauce after the simmering time, folding the meat into the sauce with a wooden spoon. Bring back to a short boil again (adding a bit of water if necessary to keep everything moist but not sloppy), then turn down to a low simmer for at least 30 minutes for savory, tender barbecue-beef-buff-pork-turk or what-have-you.

You could also place the Q sauce and meat in a slow cooker set on high for about 4 hours, and let it do its own thing. Any way you choose, the 'que will taste awesome, especially accompanied with the following lemony slaw:

. . . .

Apple and Cabbage Slaw

½ lemon

1 small apple, cored and peeled

¼ wedge small cabbage

1 carrot, trimmed and peeled

Quick shake of cinnamon — just a dusting

Pinch of sugar, to taste

Salt and pepper

Grate lemon zest off the lemon half into a medium bowl, then squeeze juice into the same bowl, removing seeds. Grate apple into bowl and toss with lemon juice. On a cutting board, very thinly slice the cabbage and add to bowl with the lemon juice and apple. Grate carrot into bowl, tossing again, then add the cinnamon, sugar, salt, and pepper to taste. Salad is complete! Makes about 2½ cups.

You know, you could check out "B is for Brötchen" on page 83 and totally wow everybody with this meal, I mean really . . .

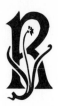

is for Roses—
*"scattered at the
feasts of Flora …"*

I intended to write all about roses. I
intended to offer general descriptions
of species roses, modern roses, Old
World types, and native species.
Then I realized I would be taking on a
monumental project, much too broad
for the scope of this book. Besides,
there are already a great many books
on roses, and my knowledge is fairly
minimal concerning rose culture. I
really do strive to write about what I
know, what I've experienced. So the tone of the chapter is altered from
the original idea.

But I'm still writing about roses. However, since you likely know
what a rose looks like (and smells like), I won't bother you with a
description; you can ogle the nursery catalogs for kicks. Instead, and
in honor of the Roman goddess of all things flowery, I'm going to tell
you about some of the ways roses are used for physical and spiritual
healing and for culinary delight.

Can You Really Eat Roses?

As long as they're not dusted or sprayed (why do people use such poisons?) or planted down the median strip of a busy boulevard, all rose petals are safe to consume. Some roses are more fragrant than others; modern hybrids, bred for color and form, are hardly scented at all—go figure! Anyway, most recipes using rose petals for food will tell you to snip off the whitish base of the petal to remove any bitterness, but if I'm using rose petals for cosmetic purposes, I don't bother with this step. When I made rose petal syrup, I snipped a whole quart of these dainties, and it seemed like more trouble than it was worth. It's a good idea to pick out the ants and spiders though; I have found gorgeous spiders among rose petals—some a creamy white color, others a pale celery green. Although spiders are my friends, I do not want them in my food or on my body. I've seen some gruesome-looking spiders while living in Florida—these babies were pan-sized! But I digress...

The delightfully fragrant roseberry tea (see page 266 in "T is for Tea") goes well with hot biscuits spread with butter and the following easy-to-make confection.

. . . .

Rose Petal Honey

Gently press 1 pint cleaned rose petals into the bottom of a saucepan. Pour room-temperature honey into the pan to cover the petals, about 2 cups honey or more if necessary, and slowly heat over low until the honey is just warm, a few minutes only; too much heat destroys the healthful enzymes. Put this sticky mixture into a clean jar and close tightly. Store at room temperature for about 2 weeks to allow the flavors to meld. Reheat honey again over low heat by placing the jar in a small pan of water (like a double boiler); after it softens, strain out the petals and recap immediately. You could also start over again and make a batch of double-infused honey for more flavor. This recipe can be used with any number of edible flowers—see page 134, "F is for Flowers," for ideas. If you have the time and inclination, you could heat the honey in its jar in the warm sun for these procedures.

Red rose petal honey was once an official United States Pharmacopeia remedy for sore throats. I'll bet it has a lot fewer side effects than all those OTC remedies.

In addition to rose petal honey, you might try your hand at jam. Since I have never made it, I'll refer you to *Stalking the Healthful Herbs* by Euell Gibbons, who offers an easy recipe for freezer jam. Says Gibbons, "I have tried many other recipes for rose petal jam, but this one is easily the best of them all." He then goes on to mention hot biscuits and crepes as a useful repository for this jam. I recall a plant identification class I gave for some homeschoolers and their moms, where we served elderflower fritters dipped in this beautiful jam, given as a gift by a neighbor, with a taste invoking heaven on earth; the kids and I picked a bunch of wild greens for salad too, but that's another story.

Gibbons also offers an ingenious method for distilling your own rose flower water. If you'd rather buy it (usually a product of France, Bulgaria, or Lebanon), you'll find that it's used in the kitchens of many Middle Eastern cooks as a flavoring, in much the same way as vanilla extract is used. Another yummy way to use rose water is in a peach-yogurt smoothie. What follows is a recipe for a delicate cookie featuring rose flower water.

· ·

Rose-Almond Cookie Drops

½ cup butter (1 stick)

⅓ cup sugar (powdered sugar makes them crispier)

1 egg

¼ cup ground almonds

¾ cup unbleached or whole wheat pastry flour

A pinch of salt

1 teaspoon rose flower water

Pinch of ground mace or cardamom

Preheat oven to 375 degrees. Blend butter and sugar until smooth. Add egg, mixing well. Blend the almonds, flour, and salt in a separate bowl, then add to butter mixture; finally, add the rose water and spice. Drop well apart by half-teaspoonfuls on a greased cookie sheet. Bake for 10–15 minutes. Let them sit a couple of minutes before removing to a rack to cool. Makes about 1½ dozen.

Good on the Outside, Too

Rose flower water is frequently used for cosmetic purposes. Diluted with distilled water one part to five, it can be used as a soothing eye wash. On the skin, plain undiluted rose water is astringent and moisturizing. Combined with a bit of vegetable glycerin, it offers emollient and humectant properties. In reference to the skin, astringents tighten the pores and emollients soothe and soften; humectants preserve moisture content.

Another method of preserving the fragrance and healing properties of rose petals is to make a vinegar extract (see page 277, "V is for Vinegar," for step-by-step procedures). Apple cider vinegar is in and of itself a healthful food, and it is antiseptic to some microorganisms. The following extract is very easy to make, and you can add other botanicals that might be available at the same time.

. . . .

Rose Petal Vinegar

Pick a full pint of fresh rose petals (mid- to late morning is the best time to pick; the dew has dried and the fragrance is coming on). You may also wish to include small amounts of these extras: plantain leaf, heal-all herb, strawberry leaf and/or fruit, chickweed, comfrey leaf and/or root, elder flowers, and/or a few red clover blossoms. After you've picked and sorted, pack these botanicals into a clean quart jar and slowly pour room-temperature vinegar over this to cover completely. I usually use apple cider vinegar, but plain white vinegar will also work. Cover the jar first with waxed paper and then the lid in order to avoid corrosion with the metal. Be sure to label and date. Shake well, and set in a window to steep. Shake every day for 10 to 14 days, after which time you can strain out the soggy herbs and put them in the compost. I usually strain through cloth to get all the particles out (do not squeeze); you could also use a coffee filter, although this could take a while. Decant into a pretty bottle and label.

I use this vinegar as a skin freshener on my face, a body splash in the shower (the vinegar smell dissipates, friends), on my hair, or in a bath or foot soak, which is very softening to the skin. Women can use it as a vaginal douche, diluted to a ratio of 1 tablespoon vinegar to 1 quart water (you best be sure the vinegar is well strained). This combined flower and herb vinegar is very soothing when added to the children's evening bath after a hard day's play. It can be diluted with water and used as a body wash during illness or fever, and soaked on a soft cloth and laid to the forehead to help ease a headache, especially if you're overheated.

Back to beverages—if you make the above recipe with cider vinegar and just the rose petals, you can use it to make a refreshing glass of rosy-ade. In a tall glass, dissolve a pinch or two of sugar in 2 tablespoons rose vinegar, then finish off with plenty of ice and water to fill the glass; very refreshing. There are several recipes using rose petals (and even the leaves) for making wine and liqueur. I expect the bouquet would be fascinating and unique. The bibliography lists several books with reference to herbal wines and liqueurs.

Returning to rose cosmetics, the following recipe for a fragrant body splash is adapted from one found in *The Encyclopedia of Herbs and Herbalism*, edited by Malcolm Stuart.

"Ancient" Spice Perfume

> 2 cups (1 pint) rose water (I see no reason why you couldn't make a rose petal infusion)
>
> ½ ounce whole cloves

5 bay leaves

2 cups white wine vinegar

Combine all ingredients in a non-corrosive saucepan, and simmer for a few minutes. Place hot liquid and spices in a quart jar and cool for about 20 minutes. Next, cover with waxed paper and then the lid. Shake the jar every few days and steep for 6 weeks. Strain thoroughly, and use as for any other type of body splash. It also makes a good aftershave—yes, guys, it's okay to smell like roses with your Old Spice. We love it.

Dried rose petals are often a main ingredient in potpourri, and are also used in herbal sleep or dream pillows (see "X is for Xanadu," page 294). The leaves of wild roses are fragrant, too, and can also be used in these pillows. Rose leaves have been used in healing poultices on wounds, and the petals have even been used in blending tobacco snuff.

These are certainly not all the ways you can enjoy and appreciate roses. There are hundreds of literary and poetic references to roses, some of which are explored in *The Symbolic Rose* by Barbara Seward. There is a wonderful guided meditation involving rose imagery called "The Golden Wedding Garment" found in *How to See and Read the Aura* by Ted Andrews.

Do the Hippy-Hippy Shake

Rosehips are the fruit of the rose plant. They are somewhat egg-shaped or rounded and can be as small as your kid's pinky fingernail or large as your own thumbnail, depending upon the species; they are red when ripe. All rosehips are edible and safe, providing they're not sprayed, etc. The hips of the hardy Rugosa rose are large and brilliant, and they are known for their high vitamin C content. Rosehips ripen in the fall, and the best time to pick rosehips for food purposes is after a light frost, which sweetens them up a bit. If you intend to dry them in a basket for future use, try to get them before the frost, and be sure to keep them in a single layer with plenty of air circulation. You may, in fact, find it necessary to cover them with a piece of cheesecloth, since I have witnessed the gross surprise (and heard this from others as well) of mistaking a maggot for a rose seed, only to discover the whole yukky thing was crawling with them ...*uggh* (and the chickens went wild)! Perhaps a food dehydrator would help, and I recommend splitting the hips in half so they don't get too hard on the outside before the inside dries as well.

. . . .

A Simple Rosehip Tea Blend to Enjoy During Winter

Take 1 cup dried rosehip pieces, ¼ cup dried lemon balm leaves, and ½ teaspoon ground cinnamon. Mix in a jar, and use 1 teaspoon to a teacup of boiling water; steep 15 minutes, strain, and sweeten with honey if desired.

The following chilled soup recipe has its origins in Scandinavia, where fresh fruit is esteemed and cherished. It is adapted from a similar recipe found in the perennial classic *Joy of Cooking* by Irma S. Rombauer.

. . . .

Rosehip Soup

Crush 2 cups fresh, cleaned rosehips (no brown petals) in a stainless steel or enameled pan, and cover with 1 quart water. Bring to a boil, then put on a low simmer, covered, for about 45 minutes. You will want to stir and mash the fruit around some during this time. Strain carefully into another saucepan. Add enough orange juice to return the liquid to 1 quart (you could also use other juices such as apple or raspberry). Mix 1 tablespoon cornstarch with a bit of the juice and about ¼ cup sugar, or to taste. Add to saucepan and simmer, stirring often, until the mixture thickens, just a few minutes, then remove from heat. Chill thoroughly and garnish with a dab of yogurt or sour cream and toasted, slivered almonds. For variety, you could add a little pinch of cinnamon or cardamom toward the end of the initial simmering time.

For a sweet rosehip syrup, follow the procedure in "The Kitchen Apothecary" under the section Herbal Syrups and Elixirs on page 14.

I'm sure you will find many decorative and charming uses for the following crafty idea. And remember, if you're ever hungry, you can always eat your necklace.

. . . .

The Original Love Beads

Create them with rosehips. First, pick enough hips to fill a large soup bowl. Second, be sure there are no thorns or spines on them, and clean off any remnants of sepal and flower (brown leafy stuff). Third, with a heavy thread (some folks use fishing line) and large sharp needle, carefully string the hips, one at a time, onto the thread, loosely tying off the end. Don't bunch them too close together, but be sure to take into consideration that they will shrink a little, so make sure the strand will be long enough to fit around your head. Hang the string of rosehips near a wood stove or other warm place to dry. Once they do, you can pull the string a little tighter so there are no spaces between the hips. Alternatively, you could use glass beads or other spacers between the hips when stringing them from the start to create an unusual original piece. If you make the string extra long, you can use it as a decorative garland and string other twigs, cones, and sturdy leaves randomly between the hips—very pretty and very groovy.

It is my intention, through presenting this information, to give you something to look forward to each spring—and fall. Having these rose recipes on hand for when the flowers bloom and their fruits ripen will give you ample time, I hope, to prepare for the busy season ahead. So enjoy, and watch out for those spiders.

(By the way, the title quote comes from Mrs. M. Grieve in her classic compendium *A Modern Herbal*, in reference to the ancient Roman festival of Floralia, honoring the goddess Flora.)

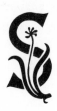

is for Sage —
the venerable one

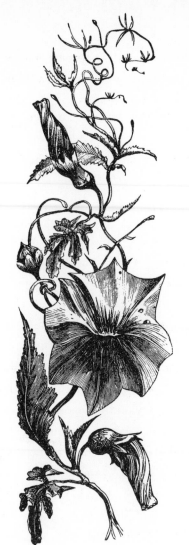

The common garden sage is an herb of great standing. Associated with wisdom and longevity, sage could be considered the inspiration for the Vulcan farewell, "Live long and prosper," from *Star Trek*, my favorite TV show; it certainly wasn't the Romulans'.

What's in a Name?

Let's not confuse garden sage (*Salvia officinalis*) with the wild sagebrush of the American west (*Artemisa tridentata*). While they're both called sage, they are completely different species. Sagebrush leaves are toothed at the very tip of the leaf, and the species name *tridentata*, or three-toothed, indicates this description; there are other species, but this is the most common. To make matters more confusing, there are actually wild *Salvias* out West too, especially in California, but we will limit our discussion to the "safe" sage, which is what the Latin word *salvus* means. Like the wild sages, garden sage (which is actually a member of the mint family) can also be bundled up into a smudge stick and burned to clear negative energy and bring about a sense of calm. Yes, the common garden sage has a lot to offer.

Sage as Nurturer

Sage has many uses in the kitchen apothecary. Besides taking a simple sage tea for mild anxiety and the occasional down-in-the-dumps feeling, sage tea can also help relieve menopausal symptoms such as hot flashes and night sweats. Boil 1 pint water and steep with 1 rounded teaspoon sage leaf for 10 minutes; strain and serve lightly sweetened if desired. Nursing mothers use sage tea to dry up breast milk when weaning a baby. However, you should avoid sage tea if you are pregnant or if you have high blood pressure. If your depression becomes chronic or severe, please do not hesitate to speak to another person you consider venerable and wise (in other words, someone sage), who can guide you to workable options, because there is no reason to suffer alone.

Keep It in Stock

Sage tea can be used as a gargle for sore throat and laryngitis, and as a mouthwash for thrush—do not sweeten. The natural volatile oil in sage leaf is antiseptic and kills bacteria and fungus, but do not use the powerful sage essential oil externally without proper dilution, and never use it internally. A strong tea wash for home use (cleaning) can be made instead—just make it stronger than for beverage tea, and do not drink. You may ask, if essential oils are so potent, why are they even available? Well, they have clinical, industrial, and therapeutic value when used properly, and this requires a wee bit of safety protocol. Sure, you can add a few drops to the water bucket for mopping the floor, but you should wear gloves if you'll be washing walls so you don't stick your hands in the water. The first protocol in safety is common sense.

To make a fragrant aftershave and bath splash, take a combination of fresh or dried sage and lavender leavess—enough to fill half of a 1-pint jar—cover with prepared witch hazel, then cover with waxed paper and the lid. Label and date, and infuse for 2 weeks. Do not drink!

A strong sage tea also makes an excellent final rinse for gray or silver hair, or dark hair in general. It adds a wonderful sheen. Check out "L is for Lustrous Locks" on page 197 for other ways to use sage on your hair.

And Then Some

Breakfast sausage wouldn't be the same without a hefty pinch of rubbed sage in the seasoning blend. And for some, roast turkey means bread stuffing flavored with celery and sage, with gravy on everything. Sage is delicious and appropriate with rich foods such as pork and poultry. You can even tie a bunch of sage to a sturdy chopstick and use it like a brush to baste foods roasting in the oven. Check out the recipe in "G is for Greens for Beans," page 153, for a tasty herbal blend that includes sage and is used to season a pot o' beans.

The Best for Last

There are hundreds of varieties of ornamental plants bearing the name salvia that are very popular in the flower garden; their square stems reveal their relation to other members of the mint family (all mints have square stems, but not all square-stemmed plants are mints). Salvia flowers are spirelike, give vertical dimension to annual plantings, and usually come in bright reds and deep burgundies. Our venerable garden sage is a woody perennial that stays green late into fall and greens up early in the spring. It can grow quite large, perhaps 2 to 3 feet high and wide, in a good location. There are many varieties of garden sage, such as purple, golden, variegated, wide leaved, bumpy leaved, large and small, but plain old sage is the longest-lived and most dependable. It sends out long spikes of lavender-colored flowers that are very charming when cut and placed in an assemblage of tiny antique bottles. I have one sage plant that is over eighteen years old and has been moved several times; I finally placed it near a flowering cherry (which has yet to flower) and other perennial herbs, and it's there for the duration, for now. Garden sage makes a beautiful component in an herbal wreath. This year I started some from seed, which I have never done before, and the seedlings are doing well and look quite sage-y in spite of their youth.

There is a tall, beautiful red-flowered version of sage called pineapple sage (*S. elegans*), and its sometimes-variegated leaves definitely smell like pineapple; you can use it sparingly in the kitchen, perhaps in a spicy stir-fry, relish, or with cottage cheese. Pineapple sage has also been added to grape jam as a flavor interest. It is lovely in cut flower arrangements. The biennial clary sage (*S. sclarea*) is deeply and complexly fragrant, and has strangely unique flowers. Clary sage mixed with elderflower has historically been used to flavor wine. The essential oil of clary sage is used in aromatherapy to balance and calm the emotions; it is also considered an aphrodisiac. This plant takes up a bit of space (but not as much as garden sage), and it sends out lots of babies if you give it what it likes, which is a sunny location, well-drained soil, and a once-a-year feeding; too much nutrition and you'll get all leaf and little flowering, which is true for all ornamental salvias.

Even a young sage plant looks wise. They are easy to grow and can be placed in a permanent setting, perhaps near a sundial, toad cottage, or garden gnome—someplace where you will stop and spend time with it, and wait for it to share some of its quiet strength in this fast-moving world. Get off the merry-go-round, plant some sage!

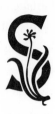 is for Sorrel Soup—
a tasty way to chill out

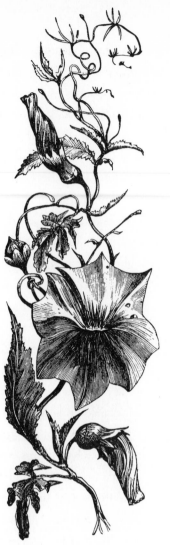

This recipe features herbs and veggies that are known for their cooling flavors. While delicious on its own, try serving this soup with grilled fish or shrimp along with a nice French loaf to dab up all the goodness.

Related to rhubarb and buckwheat (see "K is for Kasha," page 182), and to the wild salad green called sheep sorrel (see "W is for Weeds in the Salad Bowl," page 291), garden sorrel is a prolific hardy perennial with large, succulent arrow-shaped leaves and a tart flavor that is traditionally one of the early greens of summer. If you keep it well watered and shaded during the heat of the day, there will still be some growing when your cukes start producing. Garden sorrel (*Rumex acetosa*) and its close cousin French sorrel (*R. scutatus*) can be used interchangeably; they are commonly confused—except by the French, who apparently like their lemony-tart leaves less vigorous.

Salad burnet is a lovely, delicate-looking perennial that grows in bunching mounds; it makes an interesting landscape feature. While I do use it in early spring salads, the leaves are a bit tough, so it is put to good use in a dish such as this, where it will be blended into the soup, adding its own somewhat cucumber-y flavor. If you give this pretty plant a crew-cut every now and then, the leaves will stay more on the tender side.

The same with the borage leaf—it too is reminiscent of cucumbers, so it just has to be included, but the leaves are kind of bristly, so I usually roll it up and slice it super-fine when using it raw. Its edible blue flowers are a splendid garnish.

. . . .

Sorrel Soup

1 tablespoon butter

3 scallions, thinly sliced

1 clove garlic, minced

1 large cucumber, peeled, seeded, and chopped

4 cups chicken broth

1 bunch sorrel, well washed and torn into pieces
   (a bunch is how much your hand fits around)

1 borage leaf, chopped

13 sprigs salad burnet, leaves stripped from the stem

½–¾ cup heavy cream

Salt and pepper

Borage flowers or snipped chives for garnish (or both)

Melt butter in saucepan over medium heat, and add scallions to soften; then add the garlic, but do not let it brown. Next, add the cucumber and chicken broth. Bring to a boil, toss in the sorrel, borage, and salad burnet, and turn down the heat to a bare simmer. Cook until the cucumber has softened, about 15 minutes. Remove from heat.

Let the mixture cool a bit, and then place all the ingredients into a food processor or blender and whir until smooth; you may have to do this in two batches. There will still be little green flecks in the mixture; if this bothers you, then strain the soup. Stir in the cream (adjusting the amount to the texture you prefer) and mix well. Add salt and pepper to taste. Chill thoroughly, and garnish at serving time.

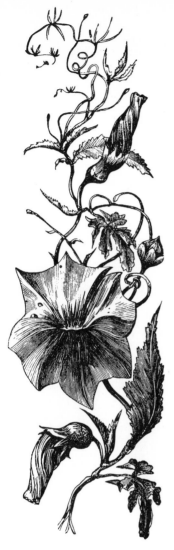

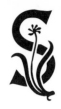

is for Spice Rack
Remedies

The herbs and spices we use for seasoning our food have long been used for their healing properties. We seldom realize that some of the food-spice combinations we consider classic are actually remedies or preventatives themselves.

Generally, the aromatic spices and seeds are used as digestive aids, while the herbs are used for their antiseptic properties. Compiled here are common seasonings and examples of how they have been used to treat common conditions. You might try these remedies yourself when the need arises. Follow the instructions for making teas (and hair rinses, etc.) in "The Kitchen Apothecary," beginning on page 3. If making tea for children, dilute it with water by half, and remember, no honey for infants.

ANISE SEED crushed and warmed in milk and taken with a bit of honey will help you get to sleep. Anise seed, sometimes spelled aniseed, makes a good tea for a colicky baby. Anise seed aids digestion.

BASIL relieves nausea and headache—bring on the pesto. A nursing mother can drink basil tea to relieve her baby's gas. Mildly antiseptic.

BAY LEAF can be used in salves and body washes. A general tonic, especially for the digestive organs.

CARAWAY soothes the digestive tract (a good idea with pastrami on rye), and the tea helps eliminate gas. For babies, soak the seeds several hours or overnight in cold water, then strain; you might want to keep this on hand if your baby is colicky, since it takes so long to prepare.

CAYENNE is a general tonic and stimulant, and it helps build resistance to colds. It's good in soup or broth to help heal sore throats. It is said to be soothing to the stomach, and folks in the tropics use cayenne, often on fresh fruit, to cool off—this is because it induces perspiration.

DILL SEED tea is used to promote milk in nursing mothers. Dill is good for all digestive problems, especially for babies (mild tea, made as for caraway), and it is said to be good for insomnia—use the leafy fronds in sleep pillows; however, I don't think eating dill pickles counts as a sleep remedy.

FENNEL SEED is made into a tea and used as a gargle to relieve cough, and is expectorant (helps bring up mucous). The tea is also good for stomach ache.

GINGER ROOT tea—3 or 4 thin slices in 1 pint (2 cups) water, and simmered for about 10 minutes—is good for alleviating cold symptoms; its warming properties will produce sweating. Said to alleviate menstrual cramps, a mild tea can be used as a compress and placed over the abdomen or lower back. Taken preventatively, ginger root capsules are very good for motion sickness. Ginger tea has been used for hangovers. There are whole books about the uses of ginger, from ancient times to modern.

MARJORAM in a mild tea is used for its calming effects; indeed, simply smelling the fresh herb has this effect on me.

NUTMEG powder improves digestion in a pinch, not to mention it tastes great in fresh eggnog. Hearkening back to the old hippie days, anyone looking for a natural high using nutmeg will be sorely disappointed; a terrible pounding, nauseating headache will result.

OREGANO tea made out of the flowers is said to help relieve nausea—just bring me a pizza instead. It is sometimes used in sleep pillows. A soft cloth dipped into a strong brew, then wrapped around the neck, is said to help remedy a sore throat.

PARSLEY leaf is very high in vitamins A and C. This herb is helpful for bladder irritation when made as a tea.

ROSEMARY tea makes a good mouthwash, as well as an antiseptic wash for wounds. The Chinese have used rosemary, sage, and peppermint as a combination headache remedy. A strong tea made from rosemary leaves is good scalp rinse and an invigorating bath as well.

SAGE tea is said to decrease the flow of breast milk; let the tea cool off and take 1 tablespoon at a time throughout the day. Honey-sweetened sage tea is used for a sore throat. Sage is another good hair rinse, especially for dark or gray hair.

THYME is very beneficial in steam facials. A simple tea of thyme herb is used for bronchial ailments.

Please note that none of these remedies are to be taken as medical advice. It is your responsibility to seek competent health and medical advice, which also means educating yourself and asking your doctors a lot of questions. Ancient healers and even modern practitioners may have used these remedies with success, but no one can foresee individual reactions or sensitivities. In any case, use common sense. Sometimes, less is enough.

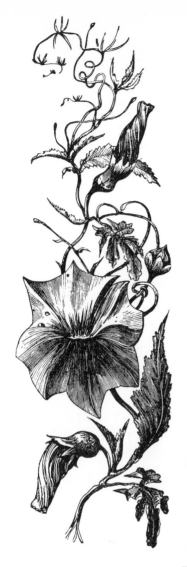

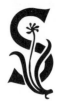

is for Sumerian
Flat Bread

Considered one of the first settled
societies in the world, the Sumerians
lived in the very cradle of Western
civilization, the delta of the Tigris
and Euphrates Rivers, in what is
now southeastern Iraq. Part of the
larger Mesopotamian culture but
speaking a language unique unto
itself, the Sumerians developed
the world's oldest known system of
writing, invented the potter's wheel,
and devised the sixty-minute hour we still
use today. The people of Sumer, or Shumera, were practical, hard-
working, and inventive. The fertile lands were intensively farmed, and
the inundation of the rivers each year brought constant renewal to the
soil—for a while. After many hundreds of years, the very rivers that
offered fertility receded and deposited ocean salts. The barley in this
flat bread represents the Sumerians' attempt to replace the wheatlike
grain called emmer (which is still found wild in the region today) with
the more salt-tolerant barley.

· ·

Sumerian Flat Bread

1 cup barley flour, plus a little for kneading

½ cup sesame seed meal (just coarsely grind some
in the blender, but don't make a paste)

1 teaspoon salt

¼ cup finely minced onion

1 teaspoon olive oil

¼ cup cold water

Whole sesame seeds and coarse salt, for sprinkling

Preheat oven to 400 degrees. Stir the barley flour, sesame meal, and salt with the onions, and then work in the oil. With a fork, stir in water a little at a time, mixing until dough leaves sides of bowl and holds together. Knead the dough, adding a bit of flour if necessary, until soft and pliable, about 7 or 8 minutes. Cut dough into four pieces, rolling each into a ball, then rolling each into a small disc about ¼-inch thick or so. It helps to roll out the dough between floury sheets of waxed paper. Sprinkle a few whole sesame seeds and a bit of coarse salt onto each, pressing in with the palm of your hand. Place the discs on an ungreased baking sheet in a preheated oven for about 20 minutes, or until they turn golden. Let cool on a rack.

According to a translation of advice about farming, Ud-ul-uru, which means "Old Man Cultivator," advised the farmers to do their work carefully and to perform "the rites" when indicated to produce a good crop. Giving thanks for the gift of grain, so basic and yet so fundamental, is good advice no matter where, or when, you live.

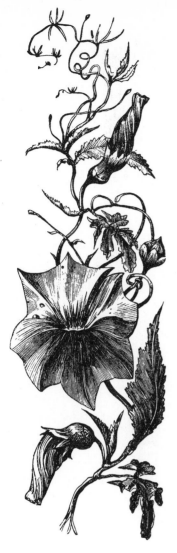

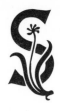

is for Sunflowers—
*and the Beatles'
theme song*

"I'll Follow the Sun," that is. It's amazing to watch the wide, golden faces turn from east to west over the course of a long summer day. While sunflowers aren't the only flower to do this, they are the most obvious. There are many ornamental hybrids of sunflower, varying in height from 10 to 12 feet tall to stubby little teddy bears, with colors ranging from warm chromatics to cool neutrals, from nearly black to nearly white. Sunflowers are a very popular and profitable cut flower at farmer's markets. This sturdy annual is occasionally self-sowing, especially under a bird feeder. The sunflower is grown extensively in eastern Europe, Russia, and Canada as well as South Dakota and other prairie states.

Evidence suggests that sunflowers are native to Mexico. The Incas in South America esteemed the towering golden discs. Priestesses wore gold crowns of the stylized flowers, and early Spanish conquistadors subsequently stole and melted down these consecrated gold artifacts. Many Native tribes in North America venerated the sunflower as well; seeds were placed on graves to sustain a loved one in the next world. Contemplative practice (i.e., meditation) suggests that sunflower seeds can be ritually eaten to seed success, as all seeds and grains symbolize prosperity and success in one way or another. With a flower that not only looks at the sun but also looks like the sun, it is easy to understand how the sunflower became emblematic of the life-giving sun itself.

Sunflowers have utilitarian use around the household and garden. The seeds are used for bird food, while other farm animals can eat the leaves. Deer will also eat the leaves; in fact, they relish the young flower heads, so I recommend growing a few extra plants and fencing in your garden (deer repellent spray doesn't hurt either; most of them are "natural" and made from putrefied eggs). Sunflower oil has been used to fuel lamps, and the pithy stalk can be used to make paper. I saved some sturdy stalks from last year to use for climbing pea vines this coming spring. Plant sunflowers in the squash mound to give the squash something to climb.

Sunflower seeds are a rich source of unsaturated fat and linoleic acid. The oil has been used by Native Americans as a hair conditioner and on the skin for psoriasis and other scaly skin disorders caused by essential fatty acid deficiency. Sunflower seeds are supposed to be good for the male reproductive system; perhaps this is symbolic, but since the seeds are so nutritious, perhaps not. Sunflower seed butter is a good alternative to peanut butter and is a good "brain food," especially for the developing brains of young children, who require healthy fats. You can take the seeds, shell and all, roast them, and then grind them to brew like coffee.

Here is a healthy and delicious recipe for crepes that are excellent filled with applesauce or sliced canned pears and a bit of fresh yogurt. Incidentally, any leftover crepes you don't eat for breakfast keep well in the freezer for up to a month.

. . . .

Sunny Oatmeal Crepes

½ cup sunflower seeds, ground but not buttery

1 cup quick rolled oats

1 cup flour, preferably whole wheat pastry flour

Pinch of salt

2 eggs

1½–2½ cups milk

Combine the ground seeds, rolled oats, flour, and salt. In a separate bowl, beat the eggs, then add 1½ cups milk. Add to dry ingredients, adding more milk if necessary, a bit at a time, to make a thin batter. Brush a small, hot skillet with a bit of oil and swirl around just enough crepe batter to cover the pan, about 3 or 4 tablespoons (make a couple of practice crepes to see for yourself). Cook over medium heat until top of crepe is dry—no need to turn over. Makes 15–20 crepes.

I grow sunflowers in my yard every year, usually the popular Mammoth variety. They grow tall and strong, with large flower heads that weigh so much I am amazed that the stalk can support its weight; sometimes they do get to leaning, especially after a good rain. They don't always reach full maturity, but I grow them anyway, their wide, golden faces watching as the bright sun passes through the sky, shining down on the garden and reaching them first.

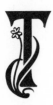 is for Tea —
the herbal kind

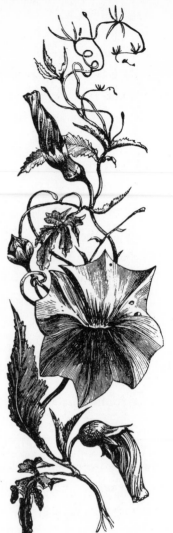

I suppose any plant made into "tea" could be considered an herbal tea, but we don't usually place *Camellia sinensis* in the herbal tea category, especially the fermented black teas we're used to, one reason being that it's specially processed (fermented and/or roasted) and contains caffeine. What I'm talking about here are tea blends made from herbs and flowers you can grow in your garden, as well as wild plants you can harvest nearby. (None of these teas are medicinal, but if you are pregnant, I advise you to ask your midwife or doctor before trying anything new, and definitely avoid the sweet dreams tea with mugwort.) All the tea recipes call for dried herbs, usually coarsely shredded or chopped, while a couple call for store-bought ingredients such as cinnamon. Use 1 rounded teaspoon (the kind you stir with) tea blend to 1 cup (or one tea mug) boiling water; steep only a few minutes, strain, and sweeten if desired.

I love this first blend, and kids like it too. The flavor reminds you of July. Store in a jar and keep handy so you can sniff the herbs to get that summery feeling any time of year—pure aromatherapy.

. . . .

Summer Breeze Tea
(makes me feel fine)

USE EQUAL PARTS:

> **Wild strawberry leaves**
> **Red clover blossoms**
> **Alfalfa leaves and flowers**
> **Pineapple weed or chamomile flowers**

Get your motor runnin' with the following tea blend, a pleasant tonic combining the best of spring and fall: roots, which are normally gathered in spring, and berries, which ripen in late summer.

. . . .

Roots & Fruits Tea

USE EQUAL PARTS:

> **Wild sarsaparilla root**
> **Wild ginger root**
> **Dandelion root**
> **Hawthorn berries**
> **Blue elderberries**
> **Rosehips**

Mix ingredients in a bowl, then store in a jar. You can prepare this tea a couple ways. The first is to let 1 heaping tablespoon herbal blend steep overnight in 1 pint water, then the next day heat it to just boiling, strain, and serve. The second way is to get the water boiling first, add the herbs, cover, and simmer on low heat 10–15 minutes, then strain and serve. I prefer the overnight method. This tea is also good cold.

I don't know if you've ever had an herbal tea popsicle, but the following blend (sweetened to taste with sugar instead of honey so it will freeze) is a good place to start. This recipe makes about 6 cups dried tea blend. If you're going to freeze the sweetened tea to make popsicles, add an extra pinch of the tea blend to the steeping jar to make it more flavorful, and sweeten with sugar.

. . . .

Roseberry Tea

> 2 cups alfalfa leaves
>
> 1 cup pink or red fragrant rose petals
>
> 1 cup spearmint
>
> 1 cup strawberry leaves
>
> ½ cup rosehips
>
> ½ cup hawthorn berries

Another good candidate for frozen pops is the following recipe. It's also wonderful made up ahead of time for iced tea, the perfect thing to sip while quietly rocking on the porch swing, listening to your sweetie strum the guitar.

. . . .

Pixie Flower Tea

> 2 cups chamomile flowers
>
> 1 cup lemon balm leaves
>
> ½ cup calendula petals
>
> ½ cup pink rose petals

Mix all ingredients in a bowl, then put into a jar for storage. Prepare the usual way: 1 rounded teaspoon to a pint of water.

The next tea blend is mildly relaxing, and the addition of mugwort, although off-limits to pregnant women, prompts the psychic dream state into play (see "X is for Xanadu," page 294). Don't make this brew too strong—steep only a few minutes. Makes about 3 cups herbal tea blend.

. . . .

Sweet Dreams Tea

1 cup pink or red fragrant rose petals

1 cup skullcap herb

½ cup spearmint leaves

½ cup jasmine flowers (you might have to purchase these)

¼ cup mugwort herb

1 teaspoon ground cinnamon or to taste

Keep the blend in a glass jar. Prepare the tea as usual and sweeten with honey, and keep your dream journal handy at your bedside.

Enjoy these herbal teas any time of year. It is very rewarding to open up a jar of fragrant herbal tea in January and be transported in time to when you traipsed through the meadow, searching out wild roses, and found bird nestlings tucked inside a shrubby shelter. Let me remind you of a few things: grow your own herbs if you can, pick only from herbicide-free areas in places where it's totally wild or where you have permission to pick, and have personal experience, a good field guide, or a good friend to show you the plants.

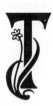

is for Twinkle Toes—
*or, my feet are smiling,
and yours can too!*

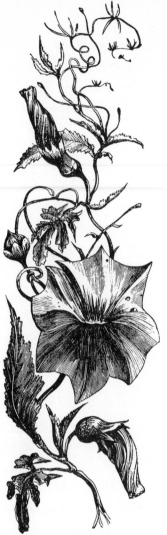

By the end of a workday, we often find ourselves ready to sit in a comfy chair, sip a soothing beverage, and basically zone out for a little while. (Kids and partners may have other ideas for us, however.) Depending on our work, different body parts may be sore or need deep stretching to loosen up. Repetitive work with the hands causes painful carpal tunnel syndrome for some; indeed, many workplaces could stand to change their scheduling and give their employees alternating activities to help them avoid such ergonomic body issues.

However, the parts that take most of the weight of any activity, and which are seemingly ignored or left till last when caring for our body, are our feet.

We must remember that our feet are very important vehicles. They are the means through which we touch earth. This suggests that the shoes we wear can either enhance that connection or disrupt it; in other words, they can make us or break us. Some people wear leather-soled moccasins so they can really feel where they are. I wouldn't recommend wearing moccasins for heavy work, though, since they don't offer much ankle support, nor do they protect the toes. I sometimes forget about my deer-skin moccasins, and when I do put them on, what a difference in my step.

Common Sense Isn't All That Common

In the classic tome *My Water-Cure*, first published in 1886, the German Fr. Sebastian Kneipp advises a regular regimen of walking barefoot as a way of enhancing the strength and vigor of the whole body, "as a means of hardening." And not merely barefoot but barefoot in wet grass, on wet stones, in newly fallen snow, and in cold water. He observed that children delight in barefootedness by instinct, "which grown-up people also would feel if the over-polished, moulded, nature-destroying civilization had not often times deprived them of all common sense." Yeah, what he said.

For feet that have been closed up in shoes too long, for gout or rheumatism, for when the body is weak or in "want of vital warmth," or "for whitlows and hurts" (a whitlow, by the way, is an inflammation around the nail of the toe or finger), Kneipp suggests any of the following warm footbaths. The first type is made with 1 handful of salt and 2 of wood ash. The second is made with 3 to 5 handfuls of hay-flowers or oatstraw. The third is made with a cup of "malt grains, when still warm," which sounds to me like soft-cooked barley. Make a decoction of one of the above by adding the amounts given to 1 quart of boiling water, cover, and steep for 20 minutes. Next, strain into the footbath tub, then add enough water so you can put your feet into it—not too hot—and soak for about 15 minutes. The original text says to cool the water to "25 to 26° R.," but I have no idea what this means.

A Wise Woman Approach

In *Healing Wise*, midwife, herbalist, and self-proclaimed green witch Susun Weed says to soak a handful of fresh or dried violet root overnight in vinegar to cover for hot, sore, infected, or injured feet, including the soreness accompanying chronic diabetes. You could also make a foot soak using plain vinegar as an additive to a strong decoction of the root. Violet contains salicylic acid, a component of aspirin. The whole plant is emollient, or softening, to the skin. See "V is for Violet," page 286, to learn more about this delicate flowering plant.

Alternating hot and cold footbaths are another method for overcoming daily fatigue and will help stimulate the whole system. The immersion should only be a couple minutes each, ending with cold. The addition of a few drops of lavender essential oil (which is antifungal), or rosemary or peppermint oil, increases the efficacy of the soak. Bedstraw (also known as cleavers), ground ivy, ground mustard seed (just a little), willow bark, witch hazel (either the simple dried bark or some of the prepared solution), and wormwood are all good choices for the footbath, especially if congestion of the upper body is involved. In fact, the mustard seed soak is even reputed to relieve headaches when used this way.

Again with the Cider Vinegar

You can use cider vinegar or lemon juice as a foot soak, the bonus being they also soften the skin. Plantain-infused vinegar has also been suggested as an addition to the footbath (see page 279 in "V is for Vinegar" for how to prepare herb-infused vinegar). I have recently had the sorry experience of gout in my big toe, a typical location. The pain and heat was horrible. First, I remedied the gout externally with a cider vinegar compress, and the relief was surprisingly instantaneous. Internally, I took a half-and-half combination of apple cider vinegar and honey (actually, heavier on the honey for taste), about two tablespoons to a glass of water. It took about ten days for the gout to go away, and this little piggy felt much better. Deep massage and breathing into the pain also helped. Gout, also known as metabolic arthritis, is caused by an accumulation of uric acid in the joints, usually brought on by excessive intake of proteins, salts, or alcohol, and not enough water consumption. Well, it *was* really hot that week ... and Joyce and Vinnie were in town, the smokies were grillin' and beer was involved, what else can I say?

Any soothing herbs such as catnip, chamomile, clover, comfrey, lemon balm, rose petals, or valerian root (just what you want—more stinky feet!) can be used as a footbath to help relieve tension. Make a simple infusion (or use a combination of two or three of these herbs) by boiling 1 quart of water with 2 or 3 handfuls dried herbs, cover, and simmer for 10 minutes; strain and pour into your chosen foot-soaking vessel, and temper with enough cold water to make it comfortable to dip your tootsies in—not too hot!

The Message Is Massage

In her book *The Complete Herbal Guide to Natural Health & Beauty*, herbalist Dian Dincin Buchman says a yarrow and salt footbath is an excellent remedy for aching feet. Follow the soak by massaging the feet with lemon peel oil made thusly: turn the intact half of a lemon inside out (use the pulp in salad dressing), place it in a tiny bowl so it can sit level, and fill this cupped half with olive or almond oil; let steep overnight, then massage this lemony oil into your feet. The author says that this foot soak and oil regimen will eventually help remove corns and calluses.

I have used oil made from steeped poplar (cottonwood) buds as a foot massage with great results (see "The Kitchen Apothecary," page 3, for how to make an herbal oil infusion). This oil is pure aromatherapy and useful for massaging the rest of the body as well. Similar to cottonwood oil is an analgesic liniment I concocted a few springs ago. The ingredients were, in descending order: birch, willow, and alder twigs and catkins; birch bark; poplar buds; and spirea twigs (the plant from which aspirin derives its name; it too contains salicylic acid). Spirea flowers can also be used, although they're not in bloom when the rest of the woody herbs are harvested. (I have come to learn that it's the eastern spirea that contains the analgesic compound, not the western, but I didn't know that then, and thankfully no harm was done. However, do as I say and not as I did—that is, get your information straight!) I placed all the plant parts in a quart canning jar and covered them with 100-proof vodka and shook it every day, from new moon to new moon. It smelled fantastic. You can either add it to the foot soak or apply it neat with a cotton pad (you might want a dark-colored towel handy, as this liniment can stain). It's immediately cooling and soothing. The liniment can be applied externally to sore muscles or aching joints anywhere on the body (except mucous membranes). You could make this liniment with rubbing alcohol or prepared witch hazel, but I prefer to use food-grade alcohol, regardless of the cost. Naturally, I didn't use Stoli or anything else top shelf, just a good mixed-drink-grade vodka.

You can also make a salve for strains, sprains, and pains. This works well on the weary feet of busy gardeners. The main ingredient is St. John's wort flowering tops (the herb appropriately harvested on a bright sunny Summer Solstice), along with plantain leaf and comfrey leaf. (Please refer to "The Kitchen Apothecary," page 3, for instructions on making a salve.) These herbs, especially the St. John's wort, are specific to the nerves and nerve endings. Massage can work wonders, especially on the feet. According to reflexology practitioners, if you consider that all the body's organs and systems correspond to specific locations on the soles of the feet and hands, a daily foot massage, even if only for five minutes on each foot, would probably help keep everything flowing properly. If you notice soreness in any particular spot, you may want to look into the corresponding body system to ascertain if there is some sort of imbalance there and work to remedy that as well.

Take a Dip

Any of the herbs or herbal combinations commonly used for bathing (see "B is for Bathing Beautiful," page 70) can be used in the footbath; just use according to the effect desired. If the infusion/decoction is strong enough, the foot will absorb the desired properties. It's sort of like the guy who ate raw garlic only to discover later that his feet smelled like garlic (is that better or worse than valerian root?); it's the same principle, only in reverse.

If you wish to really relax in the evening, if you wish to revive and energize, or if you simply wish to nurture and be kind, give yourself or your loved one the pleasure of happy feet by soaking or massaging them regularly with your favorite herbal concoction, and don't be afraid to go barefoot.

By the way, while I may be a foot-soaker from way back, I usually ignore suggestions to go soak my head.

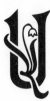

is for Ukrainian
Poppy Seed Cake

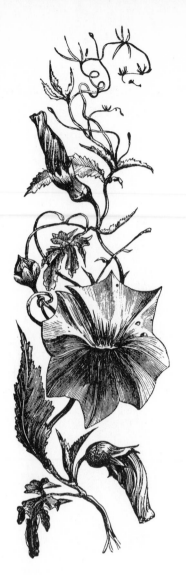

Sweet, fragrant, and rich, this cake is a welcome treat any time of day or season. Ukrainian hospitality is a well-known tradition. Also known for borscht and babka, the food of this region is hearty and satisfying.

Ukrainian Poppy Seed Cake

1 cup milk

½ cup poppy seeds

¾ cup butter (1½ sticks)

1 cup brown sugar, packed down

3 eggs

2 cups flour

1 tablespoon baking powder

1 teaspoon baking soda

½ teaspoon salt

1 teaspoon vanilla extract

3 tablespoons fresh lemon juice (about 1 medium lemon)

2 teaspoons lemon rind (about 1 medium lemon)

Preheat oven to 350 degrees and grease an angel food cake (tube) pan. Combine milk and poppy seeds in a small saucepan. Heat to just boiling but do not boil; remove from heat and set aside to cool, about 20 minutes.

While milk and seeds are cooling, cream butter and sugar in a large bowl. Add eggs one at a time, beating well after each addition. Sift together flour, baking powder, baking soda, and salt in a separate bowl. Then add to butter mixture, alternating with the milky seeds, stirring just enough after each addition to blend thoroughly. Finish with the addition of the vanilla, lemon juice, and lemon rind.

Spread batter evenly into prepared pan and bake 40–45 minutes or until done. Do not open the oven to peek or the cake will fall! Cool in pan 10 minutes, loosen sides with a long knife, then invert over a plate and remove pan. Let cool completely before glazing or slicing. The following cooked sauce adds just the right tart-sweet finish.

· ·

Lemon Sauce

1 cup boiling water

2 tablespoons cornstarch, dissolved with
2 tablespoons cold water

½ cup sugar

Dash salt

4 teaspoons lemon zest (from about 2 lemons)

2 tablespoons lemon juice (about ½ lemon)

2 tablespoons butter

In a small saucepan of boiling water, whisk in the cornstarch, sugar, salt, lemon zest, and lemon juice. Add butter, whisking constantly and cooking about 5 minutes or until cornstarch is cooked and sauce is thick. Pour over cooled cake.

This would be a wonderful cake to serve on Easter, showcasing other Ukrainian traditions such as an array of vegetable relishes and pickles and of course the intricately decorated pysanky, or Easter egg. See "E is for Eggs," page 122, to learn more about these symbols of prosperity and rebirth.

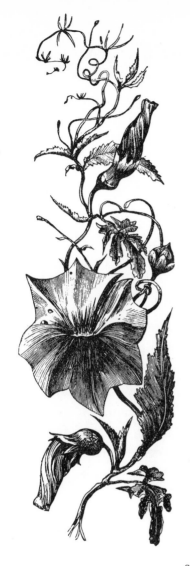

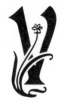

is for Vinegar —
herbal and fruited

Most often associated with the process of home-canning pickled vegetables, vinegar is a concentrated food product for which there are many healthful uses. These include externally on the skin and hair, a variety of domestic applications, and of course culinary use in the kitchen. Making herb or fruit vinegar is a good way to preserve some of summer's bounty. Once decanted into a bottle, with a sprig of the herb inside just for pretty, these vinegars also make a welcome gift. The color of fruited vinegar, in particular, is bright and stunning.

There are many recipes for the cosmetic use of vinegar. While vinegar is a great skin soother in the bath, especially for sunburn (just pour 2 cups into a full, warm bath), it is most often infused with herbs for the hair.

Internally, apple cider vinegar makes a good base for herbal cold and flu remedies; they don't always taste that great, but they do help. Maybe you're familiar with the olde-timey apple cider vinegar and honey remedies, often used for achy joints; for so simple a remedy, these are rather effective.

First Things First

According to the University of Idaho Cooperative Extension System, there are three approved, safe methods for making flavored vinegars for culinary use. However, before getting started, a few methods of procedure need mentioning. Please do not skip over this part, as I'm certain you want your product to be safe.

First, be sure to use only glass, stainless steel, or enameled containers, and stainless or plastic/nylon utensils for prep and storage (wood is not recommended, but bamboo would work); under no circumstances should you use aluminum or iron, as it will adversely react with the vinegar. Glass canning jars work great, but no matter what kind of jar you use, make sure you slip a piece of waxed paper or plastic wrap between the jar and the lid so it doesn't corrode—and it might anyway. Plastic lids work well here; I save the ones off mayo jars for projects such as this, as long as they fit.

The second step to making herbal vinegar is to thoroughly wash all equipment in hot, soapy water and rinse well in plain hot water (do not use a rinse aid if using a dishwasher). Sterilize empty jars in a large stainless steel or enameled kettle by standing the jars upright, filling and covering with clean water, and boiling for 10 minutes. Keep in hot water until ready to use. (Of course, if your dishwasher has a sanitize setting, go ahead and use this—what a time and space saver!) Sterilize the utensils, funnels, lids, and so on, as well, and if you will be using corks in the bottles, use new ones.

Third, the vinegar must contain at least 5 percent acetic acid content. This typically includes plain white distilled vinegar, apple cider vinegar, and red or white wine vinegar. Read the label; it will state this information specifically. Although they are often 5 percent, do not use malt vinegar or rice vinegar for these recipes (unless it's for immediate consumption in culinary use). Homemade vinegar should not be used, as the acetic acid content is unknown.

Fourth, pick or gather (or purchase as fresh as possible) the herb or fruit you'll be using, gently rinse any dust off if necessary, then dry on a lint-free towel. (Be careful with raspberries, as they are very delicate and can hide water in their little thimbles—you don't want to dilute the vinegar with water.) None of the recipes make large quantities; all you need to do is stuff a small bunch of fresh, clean herbs or a pint of berries into a clean quart jar.

Finally, be sure to label and date your products. Keep notes of what ingredients you've used and how much, since you might come up with a real winner of a batch. I should say that making these vinegars sounds more complicated than it really is, but you do need to follow the steps to make it turn out right.

Methods of Extraction

To make herb- or fruit-infused vinegar, read the following instructions, gather your ingredients, prep the containers and utensils, and you're ready to go.

. . . .

Basic Method No. 1

This is called "cold press," because you simply take any size jar and fill it halfway with coarsely torn fresh herbs or an herbal combination and pour vinegar over all to the top of the jar. Next, cover with waxed paper and then the lid, label, and set in a cool, dark place. Shake this mixture daily. This method takes about a month to process. After this time, take a little taste and see if it needs to steep longer. Use this method to make fruited vinegar as well, but don't shake it vigorously, just swirl it a little bit. Berries lend themselves to making fabulous vinegars; most can go in whole, but you may want to halve or quarter strawberries; cut fruit such as peaches into 1-inch chunks. I usually steep fruit vinegars for about 6 weeks for full flavor, and for variety I add a pinch or two of sugar and occasionally whole spices.

. . . .

Basic Method No. 2

This is called the "heat process" method and is similar to the cold press method, only you use vinegar that's been brought up to a boil (but not actually boiled) and pour that into the jar with the herbs. Follow instructions as for above, but wait only 1 week to 10 days for the end result. This method works well for something like spicy blueberry vinegar, but for fresh herbs and most fruits, I prefer the cold infusion. The heat process is also a good choice if using dried herbs instead of fresh (using half the amount of dried herb), especially in the hair rinse recipes.

. . . .

Basic Method No. 3

This is known as the "sun tea" method. Combine herbs and vinegar as for the cold press method, then set the container in a sunny window or even outside somewhere safe. This takes about 1 week to 10 days. Shake daily. Dried herbs also work well with this method.

For each of these methods, strain the vinegar through a cheesecloth-lined funnel or colander and into a sterile jar. You may want to strain it again through a coffee filter; this works very well (especially for fruit vinegars, which can get a little cloudy), but it takes *forever*! Even if you don't use the coffee filter, the initial straining will remove most of the particulates. You can also let it set in the jar for a day or two and then "rack" the vinegar, carefully pouring or siphoning the clear liquid away from the sediment. Put the clear vinegar into decorative bottles for gifting, and use the cloudier culinary vinegar at home for soup making—it's still good (see "C is for Chicken Soup," page 99)—or even in the bath.

Now, before you actually cap and seal your culinary vinegar, you may want to slip a perfect clean stem of herb, a delicate spiral of citrus peel, or a few berries, or whatever, into the bottle as a visual clue as to its flavoring. To give as a gift, you can tie a tag to the bottle that includes suggestions for use. Once bottled and labeled, your finished product will be a beautiful sight to behold.

Vinegars for the hair can be stored in plastic squirt bottles, as glass might be dangerous in the slippery tub. If making herbal vinegars for household use, various spray bottles and dispensers are quite handy; you can simply recycle already used ones.

Herbal Vinegar as a Flavoring

I most often use white wine vinegar for my culinary vinegars. I make raspberry vinegar every year, adding a bit of sugar to the basic recipe. Cider vinegar also works well with fruit, adding its own fruity taste. Tarragon in white wine vinegar is excellent; I love it on strips of fried calamari. Remember what I said about using vinegar when making chicken soup stock, and how it helps extract minerals from the bones? According to herbalist Susun Weed, a splash of herbal vinegar on your steamed broccoli or kale can increase their calcium value by up to one third, plus the flavor is delicious. Flavored vinegars are good on salads of all sorts, from eclectic spring greens to sophisticated fruit soirees to sturdy bean and grain compositions. Substitute herb or fruit vinegar in recipes that call for balsamic vinegar, using your imagination to determine what flavor to use in the dish.

Here are a trio of recipes for some imaginative herb, fruit, and flower vinegars. What combinations can you come up with?

. . . .

Lime Vinegar with Cilantro and Mint

Follow directions above for Basic Method No. 1. To make one quart, take the zest of one organic lime (try to peel it in several nice strips, green part only), the juice of that lime, about a dozen leafy stems of cilantro, 4 sprigs fresh spearmint, 1 peeled garlic clove, and 2 pinches of sugar. Place in sterile jar, pour in 1 quart (4 cups) white wine vinegar over all, cover, and label. Proceed as instructed above. This vinegar would make an excellent dressing over a seafood salad.

. . . .

Bouquet of Herbs and Flowers Vinegar

To make one quart, take 3 fresh sprigs each marjoram, lemon thyme, parsley, salad burnet, wild pansy blossom, and blossoming chive stems, plus 1 tarragon stem. Place in sterile jar. Follow Basic Method No. 1, using white wine vinegar, and proceed as directed. To make a flavorful sauce, dilute 2 tablespoons of this vinegar in ½ cup water and use in place of wine to deglaze the skillet after browning pork or chicken.

. . . .

Italian Salad Vinegar

Following Basic Method No. 1 and using fresh herbs, place 1 sage leaf, 2 sprigs rosemary, 3 sprigs basil, 4 sprigs oregano, 5 sprigs flat leaf parsley, 1 teaspoon black peppercorns, and 2 garlic cloves in a sterile quart jar. Cover with red wine vinegar (or use the white if you prefer), then follow the directions above.

There are many combinations of herbs and fruit to experiment with, such as:

- dried chilies and sliced peaches
- fresh ginger root with pineapple mint
- tangerine zest with warm wintry spices

…and many ways of using the prepared vinegar, too, as I'm sure you'll discover.

Cosmetic Uses of Vinegar

Plain vinegar has been used as a hair rinse for ages. It gives the hair a silky feel and shine, and if infused with herbs will bring out colorful highlights. These combinations help to restore the pH balance of the hair and skin, which is supposed to be slightly acid. If you follow the instructions given above in Basic Method No. 2, you can use dried herbs for making hair potions, which is what I usually do. Also, I recommend using plain white or apple cider vinegar for these recipes, depending on your hair color; no need to use expensive wine vinegar for your hair, and these work just fine. There are several other herbal hair treatments found in "L is for Lustrous Locks" on page 197.

. . . .

Herb-Vinegar Rinse for Dandruff

To make 1 pint, combine any amounts of at least 2 of the following herbs to equal 1 cup fresh or ½ cup dried: rosemary, nettles, mint, horsetail, violet leaf, or red clover. Follow Basic Method No. 2. Rub a small amount of the finished herbal vinegar vigorously into the scalp 2 or 3 times a week, and do not rinse.

. . . .

Herb-Vinegar Rinse for Dark Hair

Using 1 cup fresh or ½ cup dried, combine at least 2 of the following herbs, plus a pinch of ground clove, in a pint jar: rosemary, sage (especially good for gray hair), nettles, plantain leaf, red clover, and maybe even a bit of exotic sandalwood powder. Then, cover with hot cider vinegar, following Basic Method No. 2. To use, simply squirt a little over your cleanly shampooed hair and massage it in; rinsing isn't necessary, though you might want to use a dark-colored towel.

. . . .

Herb-Vinegar Rinse for Light or Red Hair

Following Basic Method No. 2, use at least 2 of the following herbs: chamomile flowers, marigold petals, mullein leaf, rhubarb root, lemon peel, and orange peel. Use the same as for dark hair.

Other ways to use vinegar as a cosmetic include a refreshing facial tonic and body splash: simply dilute it by half with water. You can sponge this wash over feverish children, or you can just add straight vinegar to a warm, not hot, bath. Infuse plain vinegar with different flowers such as rose, lavender, and elderflower, along with cooling, skin-soothing herbs such as heal-all, comfrey leaf, chickweed, lemon balm, or plantain, and use these in the bath or after a shower. See "R is for Roses" for a great rose vinegar recipe (page 243). Use Basic Method No. 1 to make these body splash combinations with fresh flowers and herbs.

Household Uses of Vinegar

Vinegar makes a great cleaning product; it even cuts grease on a messy stovetop. While plain old white vinegar works just fine, I make a three-quarter strength vinegar spray by diluting with one-fourth water and adding several drops each of all the citrus essential oils I have, plus rosemary oil, in a sprayer bottle. Then I don't feel so weird placing veggies or whatever directly on the counter, knowing I've sprayed it with a food-grade substance instead of something made from words I can't even read, let alone pronounce. You could make an infused vinegar for this use as well; herbs known for their antiseptic properties, such as thyme, rosemary, and the mints, would be good choices, along with aromatics such as clove, cinnamon, and allspice (use whole spices and not powdered). Plain white vinegar, as well as lavender vinegar, makes a good addition to the final rinse in the clothes washer, as it helps remove any soap left in the water—very excellent for washing baby diapers and blankets and so on. Lavender vinegar makes a good wash for bedrails and toys and such when the kids are sick; it has a soothing yet refreshing aroma-therapeutic quality, and it just makes everything smell cleaner (the Latin word for lavender, *lavare*, means "to wash").

Vinegar as an Old Home Remedy

Apple cider vinegar, especially the organic health food store kind, contains most of the minerals that fresh apples do, including potassium. It also contains pectin, which helps absorb mucous and some micro-organisms in the intestines; a spoon of cider vinegar to a small glass of water taken several times a day could help eliminate certain intestinal nasties. Check out "Z is for Zip," page 310, for an excellent garlic and vinegar tonic to boost your immune system.

Have fun with your herb and fruity vinegar creations. You will be amazed at the exciting variety of products you can concoct with a little imagination and only a few simple guidelines. Plus, they're so pretty to look at, all lined up on a shelf or displayed in a gift basket.

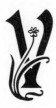

is for Violet

This little spring flower has been cultivated for over two thousand years. Most herbals refer to *Viola odorata*, the sweet violet, in all her royal purple, sweet-scented glory, but all the wild violets found in North America, including pansies and johnny-jump-ups, are edible, both leaf and flower. Since this beloved flower is so familiar, I will not give a description. The violet propagates itself by sending out runners, much like a strawberry plant, but the runners are usually hidden underground, and the violet seeds are usually sterile. It is interesting to note that a chemical in the violet flower causes a temporary short-circuit of our olfactory senses wherein we can smell its aroma at first, then we can't, then after another minute, we can smell it again, and then we can't; it's no wonder why I can never get enough.

286

Nutritious, Delicious

The dainty violet is a nutritional powerhouse, with hefty amounts of beta-carotene as well as vitamin C. The leaf tastes "green" and when young is usually very tasty, especially torn into a mixed salad. Violet leaf is also good steamed, but large quantities are laxative, so don't overdo it. Dried violet leaf, which smells more violet than the dried flower to me, makes a nice beverage tea. Be sure to supply plenty of air circulation when drying, since the leaves can sometimes stick together.

In the kitchen apothecary, a violet leaf or flower infusion is a soothing demulcent and expectorant, most often used for respiratory problems as well as a gargle for coughs and sore throat; boil 1 pint water, add 3 heaping teaspoons dried violet, then cover and steep 10 minutes, and take only half-cup doses rather than giant mugs full. Violet is taken as a homeopathic remedy for spasmodic cough. The whole-plant tincture including the root is sometimes used as a calming agent for frazzled nerves, headache, and insomnia. The fresh leaf contains mucilage and, as mentioned above, large quantities produce a laxative effect.

Soothing, Sweet, and Seductive

One of the more exquisite ways to ingest violet is to make violet flower syrup. It is soothing to the throat by itself and makes a very aromatic tea when added to hot water. The color is brilliant and beautiful. Making this syrup is one of the few things for which I use granulated sugar. From his book *Stalking the Healthful Herbs*, the following recipe is my version of Euell Gibbons' basic method:

· ·

Violet Flower Syrup

Fill any size jar with violet flowers, pour boiling water over to cover, and put a lid over it. Let infuse overnight, then strain. In a small saucepan, place 2 cups sugar to each 1 cup of violet infusion, and add a squeeze of lemon juice if desired (this is optional; the acid from the juice will make the liquid turn redder). Stir to dissolve sugar, bring to a boil, remove from heat, and immediately pour into sterile containers. Cover and label.

Besides making a sweet and fragrant tea, you can pour violet syrup over vanilla ice cream for a *parfait d'amour*, which you will no doubt fall in love with, if not over. You can also blend it with an equal amount of unsweetened grape juice and freeze it to make violet ice; just stir it two or three times during the freezing process and be ready for a most unusual dessert.

Clear Thinking

According to legends of olde, violet flowers were woven into chaplets or crowns to ease dizziness, headache, and insomnia and to prevent intoxication, while the tea was drunk to ease both heart and head. Some have considered the violet a symbol of purity and a charm against evil. In *A Druid's Herbal*, Ellen Evert Hopman says the flowers have been used in the funerary rites of children. According to Flower Essence Society literature, violet flower essence is indicated for gentle-spirit types who feel too shy to share their true warmth with others, who want to learn to trust the warmth of others, and who wish to share their delicate, sweet souls with the world at large. What would you say to little Viola if you had the opportunity? What do you suppose she would have to say to you?

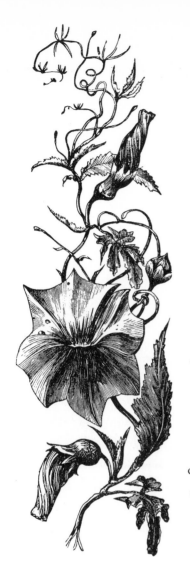

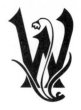

is for Walnut Pâté

This tasty spread for crackers won't freak anyone out, since there is no —*ugh!*—liver involved. You can tweak it to suit your own tastes, using pecans or hazelnuts, toasting the nuts, reducing or increasing the cayenne; or using fresh chopped herbs such as thyme.

· ·

Walnut Pâté

¼ cup butter (half a stick) — do not
    substitute with margarine or oil

2 medium onions, chopped

2 cloves garlic, chopped

2 hard-cooked eggs, peeled (as if ...)

½ pound fresh green beans, trimmed and
    cut into 1-inch pieces and cooked

¾ cup chopped walnuts

½ teaspoon salt

2 tablespoons dry sherry

¼ teaspoon ground cayenne or to taste

2 tablespoons dried breadcrumbs

Lemon juice

Melt butter in a pan; add onions and sauté over medium heat until soft; do not brown. Put into a food processor along with the garlic, eggs, green beans (don't overcook them), walnuts, salt, sherry, and cayenne, and process until well blended, but be careful not to liquefy, or it won't be pretty! Add crumbs and pulse a few more times. Taste for salt and adjust if necessary. Spoon pâté into a container and drizzle lemon juice over the surface, as for guacamole. Cover and chill overnight in the refrigerator.

Serve with a variety of crackers. Makes about 3 cups.

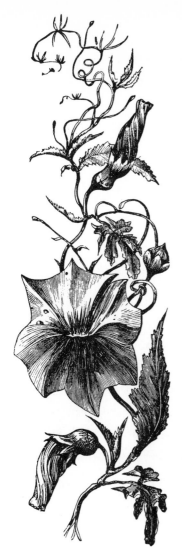

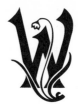 is for Weeds
in the Salad Bowl

So you say Aunt Gertrude is coming over for Sunday dinner? How about fixing up a mess of weeds for the salad bowl? Don't be surprised if she ends up showing you a thing or two, smarty.

Many wild plants are good to eat in a salad. You might want to add them to freshly washed lettuce to get your taste buds used to their unique flavors. The following are some of the most common, available, and easy to identify. Many of these weeds you are undoubtedly familiar with; others you probably know by sight but didn't know you could eat. Make sure you don't pick from places where herbicides have been used or where there's a lot of automobile traffic.

CHICKWEED (*Stellaria media*) is a pretty little plant with small, pointed leaves on short stems and tiny, white starlike flowers. The whole plant is trailing and found in sun or shade, sometimes under a hose bib or in gardens as ubiquitous weeds—it can spread like crazy and become a bit of a pest. To use, simply cut a handful of young chickweed (the older stems get stringy), wash and dry (a salad spinner is a Goddess-send), then chop and add to salads, on sandwiches, or as a last-minute addition to soup or pasta, sort of like parsley. I like to include it in frittatas (see page 124 of "E is for Eggs"). The taste is very mild and agreeable. Chickweed leaves pounded into a paste can be used as a poultice on any type of injury, especially slivers.

DANDELION (*Taraxacum officinale*) is likely the most well-known weed. I've even seen the leaves sold in the organic produce section at the mega-mart. Like your grandparents, many people still eat wild dandelion greens, and if you pick them just new in the spring, their bitterness will be refreshing. Use in salads along with milder-tasting greens or make it like a wilted spinach and bacon salad. Dig up the root, scrub, slice thinly, and add this to the salad as a great liver tonic. Dandelion root and greens make an excellent herbal vinegar (see page 277, "V is for Vinegar").

PURSLANE (*Portulaca oleracea*) is a sprawling plant with small, succulent, spoon-shaped leaves alternating along many-branched stems. It likes to grow in gardens and is available from spring well into summer. Many years ago, purslane was commonly grown and sold as a salad herb, but it is not often cultivated on purpose now. It is sour and tasty, mucilaginous but not unpleasantly so. It can also be steamed or added to soups. Purslane is similar in taste and texture to *nopales* (cactus) and is very good on tacos.

SHEEP SORREL (*Rumex acetosella*) is usually boot-high, thin, and spindly, with odd leaves that somewhat resemble arrowheads. The inconspicuous flowers turn red when mature, and you can often see soft, hazy patches of it at a distance in dry fields. Like rhubarb, to which it is related (and buckwheat too—see page 182, "K is for Kasha"), it also grows in gardens, sometimes to the disgruntlement of the gardener weeding the blueberry beds. When picked young, the leaves of sheep sorrel are delightfully sour, not unlike the domestic garden or French sorrel; in fact, they are small/large mirror images of each other. Sheep sorrel leaves are delicious in mixed green salads. The plant contains oxalic acid, which means don't eat them in very large quantities—a cow's serving, for instance—use just a handful of leaves in the salad bowl. Sheep sorrel, like garden sorrel, is also used in omelets and soups.

VIOLET (*Viola odorata*). While most people are familiar with violets in the garden, they probably don't know that violets, and their wild North American relatives, are edible and nutritious. The looks on the faces of your kids—"Flowers in the salad!?"—will make it all worthwhile. See page 134, "F is for Flowers," to learn more about other flowers you can, and can't, eat.

Other wild plants are used in salads too, such as pigweed, or amaranth (*Amaranthus* spp.); lamb's quarters, another plant sometimes called pigweed (*Chenopodium* spp.); miner's lettuce (*Claytonia perfoliata*); watercress (*Nasturtium officinale*); wild onion (*Allium* spp.); and others. Be sure to make a positive identification first, using one or more of the sources listed below and a field guide suitable for your region. Make cross references. Be sure to pick from friendly sites. Get Auntie Gert to show you too. Once you are certain, enjoy.

Edible Native Plants of the Rocky Mountains by H. D. Harrington, illustrated by Y. Matsumura (excellent drawings)

Stalking the Wild Asparagus by Euell Gibbons

Wild Edible Plants of the Western United States by Donald R. Kirk

Healing Wise by Susun S. Weed

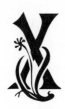

is for Xanadu —
*or, herbal charms
to inspire your own
"vision of a dream"*

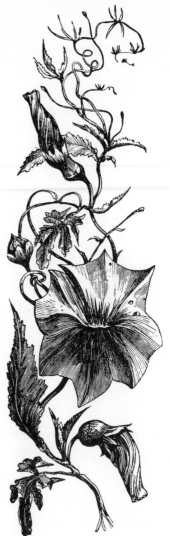

When Samuel Taylor Coleridge wrote the poem "Kubla Kahn" — symbolic, romantic, sensuous — Xanadu was his vision, a place resplendent with waterfalls, beautiful music, and all manner of exotic and breathtaking sights. Although the poet was under the influence of laudanum (a tincture of opium) at the time for his chronic pain, his poem is nonetheless a lyrical bow to nature in all her glory, a stream-of-consciousness work penned when suddenly wakened but still dreaming, as he has claimed. The herbal charms and teas I present to you here aren't nearly so notorious; they are merely intended to stimulate your inner vision without a narcotic effect. And, yes, they're legal!

Do not use any of these herbal teas or charms if you are pregnant or nursing. Mugwort is contraindicated during pregnancy. Since you are already in an altered state and are probably experiencing wild dreams anyway, it's better to wait until well after the baby is born to practice any herbal dreamwork.

Why Bother?

Why inspire dreams in the first place? Scores of research has documented that when people are continuously disturbed from sleep while dreaming, they are much less able to function and coordinate small motor movements, and become emotionally distressed much easier — all on account of not dreaming.

It is said that most dreams share a common characteristic in that they do not follow the logic of our waking thought. It is also suggested that dreams form images of what we already know intuitively. The perceptive psychoanalyst Carl Jung called dreams "the expression of the wisdom of the unconscious," and occultist Colin Wilson said dreams are the "internal universe of the mind," revealing our multifaceted natures. So, if our dream insight is more "aware" than our waking state, perhaps our dreams will contain clues about hidden issues or guides for self-development.

Mugwort and Other Dream Charms

Plants have been used as metaphysical tools for ages. Sometimes ingested for their psychoactive properties (such as the peyote cactus), sometimes used in more subtle ways (such as incense and perfume), people have often turned to herbal charms and teas to promote prophetic or clairvoyant dreams.

One of the most common dream herbs is mugwort. My favorite way to use it is in a simple dream pillow, which is a lot of fun to create.

. . . .

Mugwort Dream Pillow

Take an 8 by 8-inch square of soft, dreamy fabric (whatever suits you), face right sides together, and sew up three sides; turn right sides out. If you wish, before sewing the squares together, you could embroider or otherwise embellish the pillow with symbols you find inspiring. Next, fill it with dried mugwort leaves and sew shut. Make some sort of affirmation, either aloud or silently, as to the intent of the pillow. Place this near or under your regular pillow to inspire your dreams.

In addition to mugwort, you can also stuff the dream pillow with other herbs such as:

GARDEN SAGE—for memory

CLARY SAGE—for vivid dreaming (use only a pinch)

HOPS—for relaxation and softness

CATTAIL FLUFF—for deep memory and, well, fluff

ROSE PETALS—to dream of love

MISTLETOE—for beautiful dreams

LAVENDER—to reduce stress and promote peacefulness

LILAC—domain of the moon and the element of water,
    both connected with dreaming

You can also make small herbal charms with mugwort. Take a fluorite crystal, sometimes called a Herkimer diamond, breathe a dream wish into it, and place it in a small pouch with some mugwort to "earth" the dreams. Place this near your pillow at bedtime. The fluorite, with its double-pyramid formation, represents the great cosmic maxim "As above, so below—as the universe, so the soul."

Another dream charm that uses mugwort instructs you to take a small violet-, indigo-, or black-colored pouch and fill with a pinch of mugwort and a length of red string tied together first to form a circle.

Close the pouch, and before tucking near your pillow, enchant the charm with these words: "Charm of mugwort, charm of string, dreaming true, remembering." Pauline Campanelli, late author of the charmingly illustrated (by her husband Dan) book *Wheel of the Year*, says that rhyming helps the mind to remember, and that you should not practice these types of charms every single night, only often enough to keep your psychic channels open and your normal sleep patterns intact.

Another charm to promote psychic dreams is to take a large dried poppy head, shake out the seeds (save to plant later), write your dream question on a tiny piece of yellow paper, and slip it into the pod; place the pod on your personal altar or nightstand. An answer may surface in your dreams.

Monday is Moon Day, and the moon rules dreams. Just before retiring, inhale (do not drink) a strong, steaming concoction of three sprigs each bay leaf, mugwort, and cinquefoil; clairvoyant dreams may follow. You could also add the brew to a warm, not-too-hot bath.

Other Dream-Memory Tools

Since the average person forgets their dreams within about eight minutes after wakening, you will want to keep a notebook at your bedside, or even a tape recorder, to keep notes of your dreams when you wake up. (I'm sure there are other types of modern electronic recording devices, but I'm an herbalist, not a techno-geek.) Then, immediately write down, draw, or record any key symbols, colors, and sounds—anything obvious, repetitive, or seemingly insignificant. Use your waking senses as a guide, as well as your emotional dream-state. Date your entry, and note any of the previous day's events that might affect the interpretation of your dream.

It may take a couple weeks before dream recall becomes easier, but do not be discouraged. You are mapping your personal inner wisdom, and the symbols will gain depth over time and perspective. To value your dreams is to affirm your commitment to self-growth. Nurturing our whole selves, the dreamer as well as the awakened self, integrates us into the greater collective consciousness, which ultimately connects us to the universe.

It is said that the dreams you dream right before waking are the most useful in terms of prophecy. My most meaningful dreams often occur during the dark or new moon, while the full moon can give me crazy dreams, if I get any sleep at all. My favorite sleepytime brew? Good, fresh milk warmed with honey and plenty of crushed aniseed (strained before serving). It helps me get drowsy and protects me from nightmares, as does my snugglebunny.

Some Useful References

Aside from the fact that I dreamed I'd never figure out an entry for the letter *X*, many sources were consulted during the research for this chapter. Here are a few to help you take a deeper look into dream work:

Personal Mythology: Using Ritual, Dreams & Imagination to Discover Your Inner Story by David Feinstein & Stanley Krippner

In the Shadow of the Shaman: Connecting with Self, Nature, and Spirit by Amber Wolfe

What Your Dreams Can Teach You by Alex Lukeman

Working with Dreams: Self-Understanding, Problem Solving, and Enriched Creativity Through Dream Interpretation by Montague Ullman & Nan Zimmerman

Man & His Symbols by C. G. Jung

Cunningham's Encyclopedia of Magical Herbs by Scott Cunningham

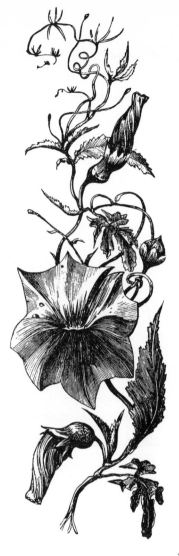

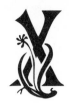

is for Xylem &
Phloem —
*or, I love it when you
talk botany to me*

No, this is not the name of the Greek comedy team performing at the New Ionian Improv. This is deep — the whole *Tracheophyta* division is concerned with the issue, and all ferns and seed-bearing plants are involved.

The architect of the original Crystal Palace in London's Hyde Park based his design on giant Amazonian water lilies. While the huge leaves were thin and delicate, they had an internal structure so strong that forest natives could place a small child on the floating lily pad and balance them there, then proceed to fish for the day's food. The leaf would hold the child as long they didn't roll around; one can only guess that after a few generations of this kind of action, the children learned to remain still after watching their cousin fall in the drink and try to climb back up. What could explain this anomaly of delicate strength?

Xylem is literally the wood in a tree—and in a water lily. This woody tissue system supports trees and other vascular plants (those plants that contain vessels for circulation of fluids); you can't necessarily see these vessels without specialized equipment, but they're there. The very word *xylem* derives from the Greek word for "wood"; the tonal percussion instrument called the xylophone derives from the same root word. Xylem is found in the roots of plants as well as the stems and leaves. The "wood"—whether it be of a spruce tree or a water lily— forms water-carrying vessels within its own structure. But it doesn't stand alone.

The phloem, sometimes called the bast, is the food-transporting vessel of the plant, making passages for rising sap. Together, the xylem and phloem form what's called the vascular bundle, a specialized conductive and supporting tissue structure. It's a complicated system of sending and receiving. Food is created in the leaves via the magical process of photosynthesis, the plant literally feeding on sunlight. The phloem is the vessel by which this food—the proteins, carbohydrates, and fats—is transported to the growing parts of, for instance, a broccoli bud or a maturing apple or a periwinkle vine. And the xylem is the structure that holds the plant up to absorb sunlight and continue the process of sending and receiving, itself a vessel of sending and receiving. What fills the spaces between the epidermis (skin or bark) and the vascular tissue is called the cortex.

The above example of spruce tree and water lily does require a bit of side-tracking here. The tree is a bit more specialized, since part of what you see, the outer bark, is not living tissue like the outside of an annual plant. Yes, the tree is alive, but the actual growing parts are sandwiched between the wood itself and the outer bark. In the very center of a mature tree is the pith—thin, watery cells that often die and become papery or spongy; the next layer radiating out is the wood or xylem (transporting water), some of which is heartwood and some of which is sapwood; this is where you can count the growth rings. Next is the cambium, where cell division occurs; then the phloem, or bast, which transports nutrition; and finally the bark, with its own distinctive layers slowly being pushed out from within as the tree expands in girth. I am reminded of the Ents in the Lord of the Rings stories and their old wisdom, because it takes many decades for a tree to mature, while a sunflower, which is very sturdy and upright for an annual plant, matures in just a season.

When we harvest a branch from a birch tree to use for herbal medicine, we peel and scrape off the cambium, or what is commonly called inner bark (and most of the phloem too), the orangey inner fiber and not the outer peeling bark, to use. In addition, we may also use unpeeled young twigs because they too have plenty of the same type of vascular activity within them. Some might call it "life force."

Imagine it like this ... water quenches your body through the supportive "xylem" of your bone and muscle tissue, and your arteries carry the "phloem," or blood, that nourishes everything, including the xylem. It's a bit more complicated than that, but this serves as a simple metaphor for the body and soul of a plant.

The soul of a plant? How can a plant have a soul? Consider the Concord grape, a willow tree, a rare orchid; but *does* a plant have a soul? What animates a plant—or anything else, for that matter—to grow and exist? Well, that is the subject for another chapter—see page 175, "J is for the Journey to the Center of Your Mind." And that is the way of us Aquarians; we can be so left-brained one minute, and the next minute we're out in left field ...

is for Yarrow

This aromatic herb has been used throughout the world since ancient times. The botanical name for yarrow is *Achillea millefolium*. Now, in Botanyworld, plant names are written as genus species—or last name first, first name last, sort of like the military. In the case of yarrow, this association is appropriate, since it is named after the Greek hero Achilles, who used the herb to heal the wounds of his warriors at the battle of Troy. The dried, powdered herb staunches bleeding, which accounts for its other names: soldier's or carpenter's herb and woundwort; yarrow contains an alkaloid that reduces blood-clotting time. Yarrow has been used among some Native American women to lessen the chances of bleeding during childbirth and to induce perspiration, but pregnant women should not use yarrow, as it has also been known to cause uterine contractions. The species name *millefolium* refers to yarrow's multi-dissected, fernlike foliage. The whole plant smells very herbaceous. For herbal healing, we use the leafy flowering tops, which are then dried or processed accordingly.

Trad but Rad

To be completely honest, although yarrow smells good as a plant, the tea doesn't taste that great all by itself. Nevertheless, when combined with equal parts peppermint leaf and elder flower, it makes an excellent and palatable combination, and a very traditional one, I might add, to remedy flu and cold symptoms. The tannin content is said to inhibit the spread of some viruses, including influenza. This tea combination, taken at the onset of a cold or flu, helps you "sweat it out." To make plain yarrow tea or the flu combo, place 1 rounded teaspoon dried herb in 1 pint (2 cups) boiling water, cover, and remove from heat; steep 10 minutes, then strain, sweeten if desired, and drink 1 cup hot at bedtime. Let the rest cool to drink in the morning. Be sure to stay warm under the blankets to sweat it all out, changing out of your wet pajamas if you have to.

Rub It In

Yarrow can be used for external care too. From a cleansing hair rinse to a steam facial for oily skin or blemishes, yarrow has also been used in the bath to relieve pain from inflammation, achy joints, and varicose veins. Salicylic acid compounds provide this action. For the bath, take 1 big handful dried yarrow and simmer in 1 quart water for 10 minutes, then strain into the tub. For a steam facial, simply make yarrow tea as above and pour into a heat-proof bowl; at the table, situate yourself with a towel over your head over the steaming yarrow brew, and steam for about 15 minutes. Freshen the face with cold water afterwards.

Fresh yarrow leaves can be smushed and laid directly on bruises as a quick poultice. The aroma from crushed yarrow leaves can be inhaled to relieve a headache—I've tried it, and it works for me. The fresh leaf rubbed onto vulnerable areas, including hats and socks, also makes a useful insect repellent. I like to include yarrow in herbal vinegar rinses for the hair, and the chapters "L is for Lustrous Locks" (page 197) and "V is for Vinegar" (page 277) each give instructions for making these natural cosmetics. Yarrow is also a component in a very special concoction called grandma's magic healing salve (see page 147), which no household should be without.

In the Garden

Naturalized wild yarrow can become an invasive weed if you don't keep it under control, sending runners under and around and sinking its roots in. However, the pretty white flowers attract tiny predatory wasps, which are beneficial insects because they eat the bugs that might eat your garden, so I recommend leaving a few yarrow plants here and there, at least on the outside of your garden beds. There are several cultivated varieties of yarrow, mostly in beautiful shades of pink, yellow, and other warm sunset colors. Last summer I planted a tall yarrow with red petals and yellow centers, a tall pink-flowered variety, and also a golden one that looks similar to tansy. I can't wait to see them come up this spring, which I'm certain they will, being a very hardy perennial. Whether fresh or dried, all the yarrows make beautiful floral arrangements. The wild plants dry to a soft golden ochre in the field, and this is a pretty stage at which to pick them as well.

And We Call Them Cavemen

In modern-day Iraq, an archaeological excavation of Neanderthal remains from the Mid-Paleolithic Age (about 60,000 years ago) revealed a sort of burial nest. In the burial site was the body of a young woman surrounded by flowers, and one of these flowers was yarrow. Many herbals mention that "witches" used yarrow for spells, but they don't say how. Sometimes called Seven Year's Love, a bunch of yarrow was once hung over the honeymoon bed to symbolically ensure a couple's vows for seven years, after which time the vows were renewed. Yarrow is also associated with the Chinese oracle called the I Ching, and the designs that the stems make when dropped from the hand correspond to a specific pattern or lesson for the seeker.

Bitter Tonic, Tonic Stout

"Wort" means "herb" in olde-timey Herbspeak. However, in beer-making jargon, wort is pronounced "wurt" and refers to the simmering malted-grain infusion—and yarrow has historically been used as a bitter in beer. One of these days, I'll talk my husband into brewing a small batch of herbal beer, as opposed to the 5-gallon behemoths most home-brew recipes make. In the meantime, I will continue to wait for yarrow in the spring, the first downy leaves appearing on the hillside. There might even still be patches of snow nearby. I will nibble these tiny, bitter morsels and know that they are just the right tonic for a balmy March day. After all, it might snow again in the evening.

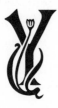

is for Yogurt Cheese

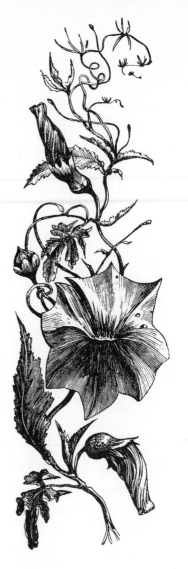

This recipe is very easy to prepare and is impressive in that you can transform it into party fare by adding any assortment of delicious bits, creating a savory spread for crackers or oven-toasted bread, or even a topping for baked potatoes. Plus, it's good for you. This recipe makes about 1½ cups.

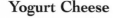

Yogurt Cheese

**1 quart (32 ounces)
whole milk yogurt**

Line a strainer with a double layer of cheesecloth or other appropriate fabric. Set the cloth-lined strainer into a large bowl. Pour yogurt into the center of the fabric. Let drain for an hour.

Next, bring up the corners and edges of the fabric, carefully twist together, and tie with a string to enclose the yogurt in a bag of sorts. Now, you must devise a way to hang and suspend this bag in whatever way practical. What I often do is stick a long wooden spoon handle through the knotted twist, then set this into and over a deep stockpot, resting the spoon across the edges with the bag hanging into the pot without touching the bottom. Let the bag hang so it can drip, drip, drip. This will take 6 to 12 hours, or in other words, overnight. While I have never needed to refrigerate this, do keep it out of the sun (which is not an issue if prepared overnight).

After this time, open the bag to discover a tart, creamy, cheeselike spread. Place yogurt cheese into a mixing bowl; at this point you will most likely want to add some salt (start sparingly) and perhaps a little freshly ground pepper. It's certainly good plain, but I like to add fresh minced garlic. Other tasty options include chopped olives (any type), chopped fresh herbs such as parsley or chives, capers, roasted red peppers, minced shallots, smoked salmon, crisped and crumbled bacon, or anything else that seems delicious and appropriate. Truthfully, I believe it will need salt or else it will taste flat. You may even wish to make a sweet spread for morning toast by adding honey, chunky applesauce, cinnamon, or what have you. I have never tried freezing it like ice cream or frozen yogurt, but it's certainly worth a tangy try.

This recipe is a good one to make with kids as helpers; it's fun and easy, and they will love making their own creamy cheese spread to use as a dip. And remember, even though it's made with whole milk yogurt instead of low fat, this stuff is good for you.

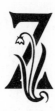

is for Zest Herbal
Seasoning Blend

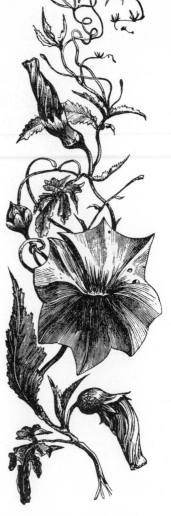

Sprightly and piquant, this blend is excellent with omelets, scrambled tofu, fish, cheese dishes, and boiled potatoes. Blend it into dressing for green salads. This recipe makes over four cups, plenty to fill a quart canning jar plus a little for your spice shaker. You could certainly make less; I used to make even larger quantities for selling at the farmer's market, as it was very popular. All the herbs called for are dried; please grow your own or buy them fresh and dry them yourself at home, as this will make the blend immensely more flavorful. This is a salt-free herbal seasoning.

. . . .

Zest Herbal Seasoning Blend

2 cups dill weed

1 cup parsley

½ cup basil

½ cup cilantro

½ cup lemon balm leaves

¼ cup celery leaves

¼ cup lemon thyme

1 tablespoon ground black pepper

1 tablespoon ground orange or lemon peel (or both)

1 teaspoon ground rosemary

Simply measure each ingredient into a large bowl, and toss them together with your fingers and hands to mix. The dried herbs should not be powdery, just crushed enough to make a nice leafy blend. I like to use a spice-shaker bottle with large holes so it can come out easily.

Zesty herbal seasoning blend makes a very nice gift. You can make a yummy dip for veggies and chips by adding a rounded teaspoon of zest to a pint of yogurt or sour cream; let sit for an hour or two to let the flavors meld. Add a spoonful of cream or milk if it's too thick.

I had this idea: what if this same blend, with the same ingredients and the same quantities, were made with fresh herbs instead of dried — what would you use it for? Stuffing a large whole salmon destined for the barbecue? Seasoning a party frittata? Nouveau pesto?

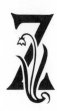 is for Zip—
a hearty garlic tonic

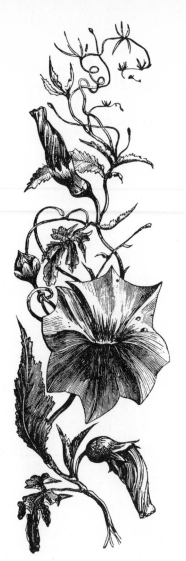

I learned about this cold and flu tonic many years ago from my dear friend Jeannine, who not only had a green thumb, you might say she had rainbow fingers. You can use zip every day in the manner of an old-fashioned apple cider vinegar and honey tonic, with the immune-enhancing properties of fresh garlic.

. . . .

Zip: A Garlic Tonic

TO MAKE 1 PINT:

Take 2 large heads of garlic (not just the individual cloves, but the whole head), wash well, then smash each clove soundly against a cutting board with the side of a heavy chef's knife (no need to peel unless they are dirty). Place the smashed garlic in a pint-sized jar and cover with about 1 to 2 cups good apple cider vinegar; use enough vinegar to keep the garlic completely covered, but it's okay if some of it floats. (Don't expect to use this jar for anything else except zip ever again.) Place a small piece of waxed paper or plastic over the jar to prevent corrosion, and then screw on the lid. Label and date.

Keep this somewhere you can see it, and let steep for 2 weeks, shaking daily. Strain, and then add an equal amount of raw honey to the garlic-infused vinegar. Place the jar in the sun to warm it, if you can, to melt the honey easier; otherwise, just shake it now and again until dissolved. You can funnel it into a clean bottle for easier dispensing if desired. Your batch of zip is now ready, and it will keep until you use it up, about 3 months at room temperature.

If you like, you can add a dried cayenne pepper or two to steep with the garlic and really boost the octane of this bad boy. I've added a pinch of cayenne powder to the basic recipe as an afterthought to take when I actually did have the flu.

To use as a tonic, just add 1 or 2 tablespoons of zip to a glass of water, and sip away. You could even use it as a pungent salad dressing for coleslaw. Your kids will probably hate it, but the taste kinda grows on you after a while. It sure does put hair on your chest.

Glossary

The main sources for the glossary are *The Cambridge Illustrated Glossary of Botanical Terms*; *The Encyclopedia of Herbs and Herbalism*; *Human Anatomy and Physiology*; *Medicinal Plants of the Pacific West*; *The American Heritage Dictionary of the English Language*; *Kids, Herbs & Health*; and *Jeanne Rose's Herbal Body Book*, with cursory glances at a few other sources, as well as Wikipedia (I have not listed each separate Wikipedia entry in the Bibliography; you can look things up yourself if you are so inclined). I have done my best to be concise and accurate within the context of this book, while at the same time make the definitions interesting. I have often been accused of serious side-tracking when looking up a word in the dictionary; I end up reading half the page by the time it's all said and done ... such a problem.

ACETIC ACID — a clear, colorless organic acid with a distinctly pungent odor that is the main component of vinegar. Vinegar must have a 5 percent acetic acid content to be of use for preserving foods.

ALIMENTARY TRACT (OR CANAL) — that portion of the digestive tract leading from the mouth all the way to the anus — the whole kit and caboodle.

ALKALOID — a group of organic substances that are usually bitter in taste and sometimes toxic when ingested. They are often of plant origin and usually not water soluble.

ALLICIN — a sulfur-based component of garlic that is available only after the raw clove has been smashed, and that contributes antibacterial and antifungal properties. Allicin is damaged by heat.

ANAEROBIC — oxygen-free, such as in the bacteria *Clostridium botulinum*, which causes botulism and grows without the presence of air.

313

ANALGESIC — a substance, such as willow bark, which decreases pain without affecting consciousness.

ANESTHETIC — a substance that decreases one's sensitivity to pain. Peppermint is a mild stomach and intestinal anesthetic.

ANNUAL — a plant that completes its life cycle, from new growth to flowering to seeding, within a single year, like a sunflower. Compare to PERENNIAL.

ANTIBIOTIC — any of various substances that inhibit the growth of or destroy microorganisms.

ANTIFUNGAL — a substance that prevents or inhibits fungal infections.

ANTIHISTAMINE — a substance that helps prevent or subdue the body's inflammatory defense mechanism to allergic invasion.

ANTIOXIDANT — a substance that prevents or slows the formation of oxygen free-radical damage to cells and prevents the rancidity of lipids in the body.

ANTISPASMODIC — a substance that relieves or prevents spasms, usually muscular spasms.

ANTIVIRAL — a substance (or process, such as heat) known to inhibit the growth of viral activity.

APHRODISIAC — a substance that stimulates sexual excitement or ability.

APOTHECARY — an olde-timey term referring to those who prepared and dispensed drugs or herbal medicines and administered to the sick.

AROMATHERAPY — the use of essential oils or other aromatics to treat emotional issues such as anxiety and physical complaints such as sinus congestion.

ASTRINGENT — a substance that causes living tissue to contract or shrink and thereby affects bleeding, secretions, and such; the term is often used in cosmetic application referring to the skin and facial pores.

BILE — a liver secretion, stored in the gallbladder, that aids in digestion.

BOTULISM — food poisoning caused by the *Clostridium botulinum* bacteria and accompanied by vomiting, abdominal pain, and weakness; botulism is sometimes fatal.

CAMBIUM — in vascular plants such as trees, the layer of cells where cell division (growth) occurs.

CANDIDA ALBICANS — a yeastlike fungus commonly found in the mouth, vagina, and rectum; when active and thriving, it can cause thrush in infants, vaginal yeast infections in women, and irritation of the intestinal tract. Proliferation of the fungus often occurs after a therapeutic regimen of antibiotics, and some feel it is responsible for chronic allergic states and autoimmune dysfunction.

CARBOHYDRATE—a type of organic compound containing carbon, hydrogen, and oxygen, and including sugars, starches, and cellulose. Carbohydrates provide the body with quickly available fuel.

CARMINATIVE—a substance that relieves gas from the digestive tract; a remedy for colic. Chamomile tea is one carminative remedy.

CAROTENES—reddish yellow pigments in plants that, when consumed by animals and humans, can be converted into vitamin A.

CARRIER OIL—a neutral vegetable oil into which a small amount of essential oil is diluted to use for massage or skin treatment.

CASTILE SOAP—a fine, mild, odorless soap available as bar soap or liquid and made with at least 40 percent olive oil; originally from the Castile region of Spain.

CE, BCE—Common Era is a calendar system used worldwide for numbering the years (BCE is Before the Common Era) and is based on an estimate of when Jesus was born; social scientists and the politically correct use this term to avoid a religious partiality, even though it too refers to the birth of a rabbi and prophet to define its parameters. (Compare to BC and AD.)

CHLOROPHYLL—the green pigment of plants, fundamental to the process of photosynthesis.

CHOLESTEROL—a lipid (fat or fatty compound) produced by body cells and required for the synthesis of steroid hormones; cholesterol is excreted into the bile. Too much cholesterol intake from foods (or an inherited dysfunction) can disrupt the manufacture of bile and cause a multitude of health issues.

CHOLINE—often classed in the B-vitamin complex, a substance that helps prevent fat from accumulating in the liver.

CLOSTRIDIUM BOTULINUM—rod-shaped anaerobic bacteria often found in soil that can cause the food poisoning called botulism.

COLD SORES—technically called Herpes labialis and sometimes called a fever blister, this refers to a small, painful sore or cluster outbreak on the lip(s) that is often accompanied by fever and usually precipitated by some sort of distress. Caused by the herpes simplex virus, cold sores are contagious via direct contact.

COLIC — an affliction that affects many babies, colic is characterized by acute spasmodic pain in the abdomen, sometimes the result of food or milk allergies, gas or other causes. Colic can be symptomatically treated with antispasmodic herbs. (The frantic parents may wish to treat themselves with nervine herbs to relieve their own tension.)

COMPANION PLANT — this term refers to plants that have compatible growth habits with, attract beneficial insects to, ward off destructive insects from, or enhance the growth of other plants. Sometimes called plant allies, scientific research is finally supporting this folkloric approach to gardening.

COMPOSITE — a flower form of the Compositae family that consists of ray florets around the edge and disc florets in the center, like a daisy, although some composites have only ray florets (dandelion), while some have only disc florets (wormwood); in any case, each floret is actually a tiny flower unto itself.

COMPOUND — a combination of two or more basic elements or parts, as in a compound tincture.

COMPRESS — a soft cloth dipped into an herbal infusion and applied to the affected area, such as a cool heal-all compress for nettle rash.

CORTEX — the tissue in a stem or root in between the epidermis and the vascular tissue. Compare to XYLEM and PHLOEM.

DAMPING OFF — a soil fungus, usually aggravated by waterlogged conditions, that causes seeds to rot or seedlings to rot at the soil line.

DANDRUFF — a scalp condition characterized by flaky skin and itching, often a result of overactive oil glands.

DECOCTION — an herbal brew made by simmering a given amount of plant material in water for a time, a method usually employed for hard, tough plant material such as bark or roots.

DEET — N,N-Diethyl-meta-toluamide is a common active ingredient in commercial insect repellent, particularly against mosquitoes. It is considered a moderate chemical pesticide and is known to be dangerous to zooplankton and some freshwater fish species. The American Academy of Pediatrics recommends that preparations containing this substance not be used on infants.

DIABETES — a disorder of carbohydrate metabolism and insulin secretion resulting in excess blood sugar and urine.

DIAPHORETIC — a substance that increases perspiration. Yarrow is a diaphoretic herb.

DIARRHEA — watery evacuation of the bowels.

DIGITALIS — a drug prepared from the seeds and leaves of the foxglove, or Digitalis plant, and used as a cardiac stimulant; it offers a more precise method of dosing, rather than using the foxglove plant itself.

DIURETIC — a substance that increases the flow of urine.

DOCTRINE OF SIGNATURES — an archaic system of diagnosis that holds to the theory that a plant will "signify" its use by its outward appearance, color, texture, etc., which is then related to the human body. For example, a kidney-shaped leaf will be useful for the kidneys, or the shape of a walnut, which resembles the brain, is thus considered brain food. Many people still use this system today, and to some degree, some of the correspondences agree.

DREAM PILLOW — this is a small, soft pillow stuffed with herbs and flowers that have traditionally been used to promote the sleeping mind to dream; the aromatic pillow is then tucked next to or under the regular pillow to gently enhance the dream state. The sleep pillow is similar except that the herbs are to help induce drowsiness and relaxation, not necessarily dreaming. Mugwort is a traditional dream pillow herb.

DYSENTERY — inflammation of the intestine accompanied by severe, painful diarrhea, often containing blood and mucus, and caused by infectious bacteria or protozoa.

EDEMA — excess accumulation of fluid in and in between the tissues, usually causing swelling.

ELIXIR — an herbal solution similar to an herbal syrup, using alcohol as an extractive agent as well as a preservative, and used for dispensing herbal medicine.

EMETIC — a substance that causes vomiting.

EMOLLIENT — any soothing or protective substance used externally on inflamed or irritated tissue. Chickweed and heal-all are examples of emollient herbs.

ENERGY — loosely defined for the context of this book, energy refers to an inherent vitality or charged state, vigor, expression, potential, or volition; everything on the planet possesses some form of energy.

EPIDERMIS — the outermost layer of skin or tissue on plants and/or animals.

ESSENTIAL OIL — a plant oil extract derived from various parts including the flower, bark, leaf, or seed, with an aroma distinct to the plant; essential oils are very concentrated, are rarely taken internally (even when diluted), and are normally diluted even for external use. They are often used in household applications. Essential oils should be used with care. Lavender essential oil has many applications in the laundry room.

EXPECTORANT — a substance that helps expel excess mucus from the lungs and bronchia. One example of an expectorant herb is mullein leaf.

FLAVONOIDS — special compounds found in many plants that, when ingested, offer the body nutrients to help fight allergies and viruses, and provide anti-inflammatory activity.

FLORESCENCE — the condition, time, or period of bloom for flowering plants. Also refers to the flower form or type on a given plant.

FLOWER — the structure in seed-bearing plants designed for sexual reproduction; flowers are often colored, scented, or shaped so as to attract insects or birds or even the wind to aid in pollination (fertilization), as well as the dispersal of seeds.

FLOWER ESSENCE REMEDY — a diluted vibrational or energetic extract of a flower's "essence" as compared to an actual biochemical extract, i.e., flower essence remedies do not contain any molecules of the plant itself. These remedies are used to relieve minor emotional issues and behavioral patterns. Rescue Remedy is a popular flower essence combination used for concerns such as the trauma of dental visits, emotional shock, and bad dreams in the middle of the night.

FLOWER WATER — a steam-distilled water solution usually derived from rose petals and/or orange blossoms, often manufactured in France, Bulgaria, Morocco, and Lebanon, and used as a flavoring (similar to vanilla extract) in drinks, baked goods, and so on; also used cosmetically as a body splash and skin toner.

FRUCTOSE — a very sweet sugar derived from fruits, sometimes called fruit sugar or levulose.

FRUIT — the mature, ripened ovary of a plant, the part that bears or contains the seeds. Fruits take on many shapes, sizes, colors, aromas, and structures, and many, to the human palate, are edible and choice. A pea pod could technically be considered a fruit as it contains seeds — namely, the peas.

FUNGUS — a non-flowering plant that lacks chlorophyll, ranging in diversity from nearly invisible, threadlike molds to bread yeast to large, edible mushrooms. Some types of fungi (plural, pronounced FUN-jee) are vital to the breakdown of organic matter in soil, while other types are responsible for severe respiratory conditions and food spoilage.

GALACTAGOGUE — a substance that induces or increases the secretion of milk.

GENETICALLY MODIFIED ORGANISM, OR GMO — has had its DNA or genetic material engineered or modified in a laboratory. Also known as recombinant or rDNA technology, the molecules from diverse biological families (such as tomatoes and pigs) may be combined to produce anticipated and sometimes not-so-anticipated results. Agriculture and microbiology are just two disciplines to which this controversial and short-sighted technology has been applied. *Author's note:* obviously, I make no bones as to how I feel about this subject.

GENUS — a botanical title comprising one or more similar species. The genus is the "last name" of the group, while the species is the individual "first name." The genus name is spelled with a capital letter and is usually italicized.

GIARDIA — a common but serious parasitic infection usually contracted from drinking water from streams or lakes (or sometimes untreated municipal water) contaminated with this protozoa. The infection usually takes a couple weeks to become symptomatic and causes severe abdominal cramps, diarrhea, and nausea, amongst other things. Giardia can be avoided by never drinking from a stream, and using a water filter on hiking and camping trips as well as on the tap at home.

GOUT — metabolic arthritis in which excess uric acid in the blood crystallizes and is deposited in the joints, causing pain and inflammation. Gout is considered to be a hereditary condition.

HAIR FOLLICLES — a tubelike opening in the skin where a hair develops and grows out.

HANGOVER — the unpleasant and often miserable effects one experiences after consuming excessive amounts of alcohol, partly caused by excessive dehydration.

HEADSPACE — in the context of home food preservation and not the above definition, the distance in inches between the lid or cap on a jar and the liquid inside; a ½-inch headspace means there is ½ inch from the liquid to the cap on the jar.

HERPES — an inflammatory skin condition caused by the herpes simplex virus, causing cold sores or fever blisters on or near the mouth/lip or genital area, although each strain can appear on either site. Herpes is contagious and very painful, and precautions must be made to prevent spreading the virus by avoiding direct contact with the sores. While the blisters can last from a few days to a couple weeks, the virus can lie dormant for months to years before some type of stressor, such as emotional upheaval, overexertion, or excessive heat, triggers an outbreak. There is no cure for herpes at this time, but lemon balm is one herb effective in treating the symptoms, used as a tincture internally and a wash externally.

HIV — Human immunodeficiency virus, which may be responsible for AIDS (Acquired Immune Deficiency Syndrome) and affects some people more seriously than others.

HUMECTANT — a substance that helps the skin retain moisture, usually some sort of liquid.

IMMUNE SYSTEM — the body's mechanism of resistance to foreign agents, or pathogens, or the toxins they release. Specialized cells (lymphocytes and macrophages are two types) recognize the presence of these agents and respond by destroying the invading organism.

INFLAMMATION — localized heat, swelling, redness, and pain as a result of irritation, infection, or injury.

INFUSION — a medicinal tea prepared the same as for beverage tea except that the amount of herbs used is greater and is taken by the dose. An infusion is a remedy; tea is a beverage.

INULIN — a complex sugar found in several plants (often in members of the Compositae family such as dandelion and Jerusalem artichoke), which is said to be easier for diabetics to consume.

LAXATIVE — a substance that stimulates the evacuation of the bowels.

LEAF — a (usually) green, flattened structure growing from out of the stem of vascular plants and functioning as the principal organ of photosynthesis. The leaf itself often has a stem that attaches to the main stem of a plant or emerges from the ground in a rosette form. Leaves vary widely in appearance, and many are edible and choice.

LECITHIN—a complex lipid or fatty compound found in all plant and animal tissues, and when consumed aids in the absorption of essential fatty acids. Egg yolk is one source of lecithin.

LIMBIC SYSTEM—a group of interconnected structures within the brain that produce the range of human emotional feelings and memory function, as well as our basic necessary functions such as heartbeat and respiration.

LINIMENT—a substance applied to the skin and used to relieve symptoms such as pain or irritation.

LINOLEIC ACID—an essential fatty acid vital to the human diet.

LYMPHATIC SYSTEM—Herbalist Michael Moore calls this the "back alley" of blood circulation, wherein the lymph, or the clear intercellular fluid that drains from the capillaries, basically filters the "junk" out of the blood and sends it back into play for another round in the circulatory system. It's a lot more complicated than that, but this metaphor serves as quick explanation for what is an amazing immune regulator. Unlike blood, which has the heart to pump it through the body, lymph does not circulate on its own but must be stimulated by physical activity.

MEDITATION—an exercise of reflection or contemplation used to quiet the mind and relax the body; often devotional in nature.

MENINGITIS—an inflammation of the meninges, the membranes covering the brain, caused by bacteria or a virus that invades the spinal fluid. It most often occurs in infants and can cause loss of vision or hearing, paralysis, or developmental disabilities.

MICROORGANISMS—a plant or animal so small that it can only be seen through a microscope; a bacteria or protozoa.

MUCILAGE—a gummy, sticky, or slimy substance found in some plants, often useful for soothing irritated conditions. Cooked barley is mucilaginous and soothing to the stomach and intestines.

NATIVE—indigenous to or originating from a certain place, as compared to foreign or exotic. Lemons are native to India.

NATURALIZED—adapted or acclimated to a new climate or environment. Lemons are naturalized to California.

NERVINE—a substance that calms nervousness and irritability; compare to SEDATIVE.

NEURON—a complete nerve cell including the cell body and the extensions, or nerve fibers, that conduct impulses.

OINTMENT — a substance of varying solidity, usually oil- or fat-based and infused with herbs, and used on the skin as a balm to soothe irritation or to heal scrapes or scars.

OLFACTORY — of or pertaining to the sense of smell.

PECTIN — a complex colloidal substance found in ripe fruits such as apples and used as a thickening agent for various foods and cosmetics.

PELLAGRA — a chronic disease caused by niacin deficiency and characterized by dermatitis, inflamed digestive tract, and mental disorders. This disease is usually associated with corn-based diets except where the corn is treated with lye or ash to make it soft (and to make the niacin available for absorption), such as with tortillas or hominy.

PERENNIAL — a plant that lives for a number of years, such as a rose bush; some perennials are deciduous, losing their leaves in the fall (like the rose), and some are evergreen, with leaves that adhere through the winter (such as Oregon grape).

PETALS — a single segment of the corolla, or ring of petals, of a flower. A wild rose has five petals around the ring.

pH — the acid or alkaline quotient (or hydrogen-ion concentration) of a substance measured on a scale from pH 1 (very acidic) to pH 14 (very alkaline). Distilled water is neutral at pH 7, human blood slightly alkaline at pH 7.4, and lemons acidic at pH 2.3. This unit of measure is of serious concern to the master food preserver and master gardener alike.

PHEROMONES — specialized aromatic chemicals secreted by one individual and affecting the sexual physiology of another; sex hormones. Pheromones do not produce a detectable scent, but they are nevertheless quite potent.

PHLOEM — the vascular tissue in a plant that allows nutrient-rich sap to move from the outer leaves to other parts of a plant. Compare with XYLEM.

PHOTOSYNTHESIS — a process wherein green plants convert carbon dioxide and water into carbohydrates (food) in the presence of sunlight. Only plants with chlorophyll go through photosynthesis.

PITH — the column of spongy, cellular tissue in the center of trees and the stems and branches of most vascular plants.

PLASTER — an herbal paste mixed with equal parts bran (or other neutral medium) and hot water, spread onto a cloth, and applied to the affected body part needing treatment, such as a mustard plaster applied to the chest to stimulate circulation and open breathing passages.

POLIO — or poliomyelitis, is a viral disease occurring mainly in children that affects the motor neurons of the spine; the infection may cause paralysis, muscular atrophy, and physical deformity. The polio vaccine in the United States has reduced the spread of polio; however, some people consider vaccinations to be as dangerous as the disease they are supposed to protect against. Considering that many of these preparations contain a mercury-compound base, it does make one wonder.

POME — a type of fruit with a woody core, seed cavities, and firm flesh attached to a stem; in particular, members of the apple and rose family.

POTPOURRI — (pronounced po-purr-EE) a blended mixture of sweet-scented flowers and leaves along with aromatic spices, resins, or roots and "fixed" with a stabilizing substance such as salt or orris root to preserve the aroma. It is pretty to look at and lovely to smell, as long as artificial scents are avoided in its creation. Rose petals and lavender are traditional ingredients in potpourri.

POULTICE — an herbal paste applied externally to bruises, scrapes, or other inflammations; it can be used by itself or spread on a soft cloth and laid over the affected area.

PROTEIN — a complex nitrogen-based organic compound composed of amino acid molecules. Protein occurs in all living matter and is essential for the growth and repair of animal tissue.

REPRODUCTION — the sexual or asexual process by which organisms generate more of their own kind; the process of making a new individual. Also indicates the process of cell replication such as in the case of injury. Reproduction is a characteristic that defines life as we know it.

RHEUMATISM — an inflammation of the fibrous tissue that surrounds a joint, causing the joint to feel tender and stiff.

RHINENCEPHALON — the olfactory region of the brain, literally the "nose-brain."

RHIZOME — a rootlike stem that lies horizontal on or directly under the ground, from which buds, shoots, or fibery roots emerge.

ROOT — the underground part of the plant, often branched or divided, that anchors the plant to the soil and absorbs nutrients. There are several root forms; many roots are edible, such as horseradish and carrot.

RUTIN — an antioxidant agent found in buckwheat and other plants, responsible for strengthening the capillaries and preventing oxygen free-radical damage to cells, which some believe helps prevent cancer.

SAFETY PROTOCOL — basically, these are the steps you take when approaching a project of any kind where you read the instructions thoroughly and gather all tools and ingredients ahead of time, and anticipating any contingencies that may come up, such as hot liquid spills (hot pads and paper towels), sharp items around young children (Gramma will chop the roots), generally planning for the safety of the those involved in the project, and doing some background study on your subject matter. In other words, it's the common sense that ain't so common.

SALICYLIC ACID — a substance used in making aspirin and also for the treatment of certain skin conditions such as warts and eczema.

SALVE — a soothing or healing compound usually oil-based and containing extracts to treat skin irritations and bruises; same as OINTMENT.

SAP — the juice of a plant or tree.

SAPONINS — a soapy colloidal agent found in various plants that make a sudsy lather when agitated with water; used in various household and cosmetic applications.

SATURATED FAT — a type of lipid or fat wherein each carbon atom is bonded to as many hydrogen atoms as possible and is thus "saturated"; these fats tend to be solid at room temperature and are usually heat stable; lard is a saturated fat. Fats are organic compounds and are vital to cell proliferation and activity, but an overabundance of saturated fats tends to accumulate in the liver and blood, causing health problems such as heart disease and high cholesterol.

SEDATIVE — a substance that induces sleep; compare to NERVINE.

SLEEP PILLOW — similar to a dream pillow, this is a soft pillow stuffed with sweet-smelling herbs used to induce relaxation and sleep. Dill, whose name means "to lull," is a common sleep pillow herb.

SMUDGE — this is the practice of using smoke from smoldering dried herbs or resins to purge or clear a person, place, or object of disagreeable energy, or to welcome desirable energy into the object or environment. It is also used as a way of sending prayers. In North America, many evergreens and sages are used as smudge herbs, either crumbled and burned in a heatproof bowl or tied with string into smudge sticks (like a wand) and lit at one end to burn until one intuits the situation is clear or blessed.

SPECIES — representing the botanical "second name" of a plant or animal (what I call the "first name last" part of this system of classification), serving to distinguish one species from another in the same genus. In this system, my own name would be thus: Shababy doreen, wherein Shababy is my genus name and doreen is my species name. I could Latinize it by calling it doreeni, but I digress for my own amusement.

SPIRIT PLATE — a highly personal way of giving thanks for a meal by placing a tiny amount of all the foods served onto a plate and blessing the meal, the food, and the participants, then placing the plate outdoors to leave for the "spirits" to use as they see fit; a way of saying grace.

SPORES — the reproductive unit in ferns and other plants such as moss.

STEEP — to soak fresh or dried herbs in boiling water (or according to instructions) for a given time, then strain to make a tea, an infusion, or a decoction.

STREWING HERB — in the less-hygienic days of yore, when goats and ducks may have shared a section of the home with humans during the winter, herbs were traditionally strewn about the floor to absorb dampness and odors and to repel mice and insects; juniper, lavender, and tansy were common strewing herbs that were simply swept up after a time and replaced with fresh herbs.

SUCROSE — a disaccharide carbohydrate found in many plants but manufactured mostly from sugar cane and sugar beets, and also used in making cellulose. Table sugar is sucrose.

SYRUP — in the context of this book, an herbal or fruit extract sweetened and preserved with sugar or honey, and used to deliver herbs that might otherwise be distasteful or to make yummy toppings for pancakes and yogurt.

TANNIN — an astringent, protective substance found in plant tissue.

TEA — a beverage made from steeping leaves or flowers of specific plants in boiling water for a given time, then strained and sipped for enjoyment.

TEMPERATE ZONE—a temperature and/or climate zone where snow falls and stays on the ground every year, and the typical growing season is about 100 days from the last frost in spring to the first frost in autumn.

TEOSINTE—the ancestor of our modern-day corn, or maize, known to be many thousands of years old.

TINCTURE—an alcohol solution of plant material that extracts constituents not completely water soluble; tinctures are a concentrated liquid herbal potion, and doses are taken in drops.

TONIC—often used preventatively, a tonic is a substance used to strengthen the system, usually in the absence of injury or disease. Grandma's spring dandelion tonic is used to flush out the system of winter's fats and carbohydrates and jump-start the metabolism into the activity of spring.

TYPHOID—a disease caused by a highly infectious bacteria, *Salmonella typhosa*, and causing rash, high fever, and intestinal hemorrhage; usually transmitted by food or water.

UNGUENT—an oil-based herbal preparation used for healing or cosmetic purposes; an unguent is the same as a salve or ointment.

UNSATURATED FAT—a fat with one or more double bonds between the carbon atoms, resulting in fats that tend to be liquid at room temperature, such as salad oil; while too much of a good thing is not good, these fats are generally healthier than saturated fats, though less heat stable.

VASCULAR PLANTS—plants that have a system of xylem and phloem to conduct water and nutrients.

VIRUS—from the Latin meaning "toxin" or "poison," a virus is a subatomic infectious agent that is unable to grow or reproduce without a host cell. Viruses can infect all cellular life and are about 100 times smaller than bacteria. The invention of the electron microscope in 1931 gave us the first images of viruses. Opinions differ on whether or not viruses are a form of life (loosely defined as organic structures that display specific characteristics such as movement, responsiveness, digestion, circulation, and excretion). Although viruses have genes and evolve through natural selection, they do not have a cellular structure or metabolism. "Accepted" life forms use cell division to reproduce, while viruses spontaneously assemble, creating multiple copies of themselves, similar to the growth of crystals. The effect of viruses on the host cells is varied and extensive.

VOLATILE OIL — those plant oils that evaporate quickly, unlike an essential oil, which is a concentrated distillation and remains potent and aromatic for a long period of time.

WEED — to quote from *Rodale's All-New Encyclopedia of Organic Gardening*, "fast, tough and common — that's all it takes to earn a plant the name of weed." A weed can be any invasive plant in the wrong place at the wrong time; yarrow growing up in the cabbage bed is a troublesome, pushy neighbor, but yarrow growing outside the raised bed is harbor to beneficial insects that eat cabbage-lovin' caterpillars. Weeds are wild and untamed, and not always in the top-ten list of raving beauties. But since they do exist here on the planet along with the rest of us, it is this writer's opinion that they have their place in the cosmic scheme of things, even if we can't always figure out what it is. Besides, wild and untamed is a good thing.

WHITLOW — an inflammation around the nail of a toe or finger. *Ouch*.

WORT — or *wyrt* in Old English means "plant." Also, the infusion of malted grains used to make ale or beer, pronounced *wurt*.

XYLEM — the vascular tissue of a plant or tree that conducts water to the rest of the plant; the structure of this tissue facilitates the phloem in moving nutrient-rich sap throughout the plant.

List of Plants
(and Their Botanical Names)

Plants are scientifically named according to a system called binomial nomenclature, or "two-name naming," so to speak; so are animals and every other known living creature on earth. This gives them a *Generic* name (capitalized) and a *specific* name (small case), and these names are usually written *italicized*. Another way to look at it is that their names are arranged in a last-name-first, first-name-last manner. Most of the words are derived from Latin, but the rest are Greek. (Truth be told, some botanical names are simply a Latinized version of the name of the botanist who "discovered" the plant.)

The Swedish botanist Carolus Linnaeus is credited with devising this system of naming, which he presented to the scientific community sometime around 1737. Each word of a plant name refers first to generic or general qualities shared within the family, then the specific qualities that make that plant an individual within that particular family. A good example of this would be the Mint family; there are many individual species of *Mentha*, but they still share enough characteristics to have the same "last name." Linnaeus's original system predates Darwin's theory of evolution, and he did not necessarily classify plants according to actual family but rather to form. Modern taxonomic classification uses an updated binomial system now to describe a plant, such as *Chenopodium album*, so it can be known all over the world by that name, as compared to the common name pigweed, which could describe perhaps a dozen other common pigweeds of different families. Personally, I still call *C. album* by a common name I learned from a couple of old geezers who roused my curiosity concerning wild plants; the old ranchers called it lamb's quarters, which has kind of a nice ring to it. Tastes like spinach.

What follows is a list of all the plants mentioned in this book — all the herbs, flowers, trees, and even food plants I have made reference to in one way or another — with their commonly used names followed by their commonly used botanical name; this does change on occasion, but then I'm still calling Pluto a planet. Also included are a few "also known as" names for some of these plants. Once you get the hang of learning the botanical names and what they actually mean in Latin or Greek, you will see the relationships between the plants a little better and be able to pronounce those spells in the Harry Potter books with a little more flair as well.

ALDER — *Alnus* spp.

ALFALFA — *Medicago sativa*

ALLSPICE — *Pimenta dioica*

ALMOND — *Amygdalus communis*

ANGELICA — *Angelica archangelica*

ANISE — *Pimpinella anisum* (aniseed)

APPLE — *Malus pumila*

ARTICHOKE — *Cynara scolymus*

ARUGULA — *Eruca sativa*

AVOCADO — *Persea americana*

BARLEY — *Hordeum vulgare*

BASIL — *Ocimum basilicum*

BAY LEAF — *Laurus nobilis*

BEDSTRAW — *Galium aparine* (cleavers)

BEE BALM — *Monarda didyma* (Oswego tea, monarda)

BEET — *Beta vulgaris* (Crassa group)

BIRCH — *Betula* spp.

BLACKBERRY — *Rubus* spp. (bramble)

BLEEDING HEART — *Dicentra* spp.

BLUE CAMAS — *Camassia quamash*

BORAGE — *Borago officinalis*

BUCKWHEAT — *Fagopyrum esculentum*

BURDOCK — *Arctium lappa, A. minus*

BUTTERCUP — *Ranunculus* spp.

CALENDULA — *Calendula officinalis* (pot marigold, marigold)

CARAWAY — *Carum carvi*

CATNIP — *Nepeta cataria*

CATTAIL — *Typha latifolia*

CAYENNE — *Capsicum annuum* (chili pepper)

CELERY — *Apium graveolens*

CHAMOMILE — *Matricaria recutita* (German chamomile)

CHAMOMILE — *Chamaemelum nobile* (Roman chamomile)

CHARD — *Beta vulgaris* (Cicla group)

CHICKWEED — *Stellaria media*

CHICORY — *Cichorium intybus*

CILANTRO — *Coriandrum sativum* (same plant as coriander seed)

CINNAMON — *Cinnamomum zeylanicum* (Ceylon cinnamon)

CINQUEFOIL — *Potentilla anserina* (silverweed, five-finger)

CLARY SAGE — *Salvia sclarea*

CLEMATIS — *Clematis* spp. (virgin's bower)

CLOVE — *Syzygium aromaticus*

COCOA — *Theobroma cacao* (cacao)

COCONUT — *Cocos nucifera*

COFFEE — *Coffea arabica*

COMFREY — *Symphytum officinale* (knitbone)

CORN — *Zea mays*

COTTONWOOD — *Populus trichocarpa* (black cottonwood, poplar)

CREOSOTE BUSH — *Larrea tridentata* (chapparal)

DANDELION — *Taraxacum officinal*

DEATH CAMAS — *Zigadenus* spp.

DELPHINIUM — *Delphinium* spp.

DILL — *Anethum graveolens*

ELDERBERRY — *Sambucus* spp.

EUCALYPTUS — *Eucalyptus globulus*

FENNEL — *Foeniculum vulgare* (seed fennel), *F. dulce* (sweet fennel)

FOXGLOVE — *Digitalis purpurea*

GARLIC — *Allium sativa*

GINGER — *Zingiber officinale*

GINSENG — *Panax quinquefolium* (American ginseng)

GOLDENROD — *Solidago* spp.

GRAPE — *Vitis labrusca* (American, "foxy"), *V. vinifera* (European)

GROUND IVY — *Glechoma hederacea* (alehoof)

HAWTHORN — *Crataegus douglasii* (western)

HEAL ALL — *Prunella vulgaris* (self-heal)

HEMLOCK — *Tsuga* spp. (the tree)

HEMLOCK — *Cicuta* spp. (not the tree)

HENNA — *Lawsonia alba*

HOLLYHOCK — *Alcea rosea*

HOPS — *Humulus lupulus*

HOREHOUND — *Marrubium vulgare*

HORSERADISH — *Armoracia rusticana*

HORSETAIL — *Equisetum arvense* (scouring rush)

HUCKLEBERRY — *Vaccinum* spp. (bilberry)

HYDRANGEA — *Hydrangea* spp.

IRIS — *Iris* spp. (flag)

JASMINE — *Jasminum officinale*

JERUSALEM ARTICHOKE — *Helianthus tuberosus* (sunchoke)

JOJOBA — *Simmondsia chinensis*

JUNIPER — *Juniperus communsis*

KELP — *Laminaria* spp., *Fucus* spp.

KINNIKINNICK — *Arctostaphylos uva-ursi* (bearberry)

LAMB'S QUARTERS — *Chenopodium album* (one of several plants known as pigweed)

LAVENDER — *Lavandula officinalis*

LEMON — *Citrus limon*

LEMON BALM — *Melissa officinalis*

LEMON THYME — *Thymus x citriodorus*

LETTUCE — *Lactuca sativa*

LICORICE — *Glycyrrhiza glabra*

LILAC — *Syringa vulgaris*

LIME — *Citrus aurantifolia*

LUPINE — *Lupinus* spp.

MAPLE — *Acer* spp.

MARIGOLD — *Tagetes* spp. (garden marigold)

MARJORAM — *Oreganum marjoranum* (sweet marjoram)

MARSH MALLOW — *Althea officinalis*

MISTLETOE — *Viscum album* (European mistletoe)

MONKSHOOD — *Aconitum* spp. (aconite)

MOREL MUSHROOM — *Morchella esculenta*

MUGWORT — *Artemisia vulgaris*

MULBERRY — *Morus rubra, M. alba, M. nigra*

MULLEIN — *Verbascum thapsis*

MUSTARD — *Brassica juncea* (seed)

NASTURTIUM — *Tropaeolum majus* (common garden nasturtium)

NETTLES — *Urtica dioica*

NIGHTSHADE — *Atropa belladonna* (deadly nightshade)

NUTMEG — *Myristica fragrans*

OATS — *Avena sativa*

OLEANDER — *Nerium oleander, Thevetia* spp. (yellow oleander)

ONION — *Allium cepa*

ORANGE — *Citrus sinensis*

OREGANO — *Oreganum vulgare*

OREGON GRAPE — *Mahonia aquifolium*

PANSY — *Viola tricolor* (Johnny jump-up, viola)

PARSLEY — *Petroselinum crispum*

PATCHOULI — *Pogostemon patchouli*

PENNYROYAL — *Hedeoma pulegioides* (American), *Mentha pulegium* (European)

PEONY — *Paeonia* spp.

PEPPER — *Piper nigrum* (black pepper)

PERIWINKLE — *Vinca* spp.

PINE — *Pinus* spp.

PINEAPPLE SAGE — *Salvia elegans*

PINEAPPLE WEED — *Matricaria matricarioides*

PLANTAIN — *Plantago major* (broad leaf), *P. lanceolata* (lance leaf)

POINSETTIA — *Euphorbia pulcherrima*

POPPY — *Papaver somniferum* (seed poppy)

PURSLANE — *Portulaca oleracea*

RADISH — *Raphanus sativus*

RASPBERRY — *Rubus* spp.

RED CLOVER — *Trifolium pratense*

RHUBARB — *Rheum rhabarbarum*

RICE — *Oryza sativa*

ROSE — *Rosa* spp.

ROSEMARY — *Rosmarinus officinalis*

SAGE — *Salvia officinalis* (garden sage)

SAGE — *Artemisia tridentata* (sagebrush)

SALAD BURNET — *Sanguisorba minor*

SANDALWOOD — *Santalum alba*

SAVORY — *Satureja hortensis* (summer savory)

SELF-HEAL — *Prunella vulgaris* (heal-all)

SESAME — *Sesamum indicum*

SHEEP SORREL — *Rumex acetosella*

SKULLCAP — *Scutellaria* spp.

SOAPWORT — *Saponaria offinalis*

SORREL — *Rumex acetosa* (garden sorrel), *R. scutatus* (French sorrel)

SPEARMINT — *Mentha spicata*

SPINACH — *Spinacia oleracea*

ST. JOHN'S WORT — *Hypericum perforatum* (Klamath weed)

SUNFLOWER — *Helianthus annuus*

SWEET PEA — *Lathyrus odoratus*

SWEET WOODRUFF — *Galium odoratum*

TANSY — *Tanacetum vulgare* (external use only)

TARRAGON — *Artemisia dracunculus 'Sativa'* (French tarragon)

THYME — *Thymus vulgaris* (English thyme, garden thyme)

TURMERIC — *Curcuma longa*

VALERIAN — *Valerian officinalis*

VIOLET — *Viola odorata* (sweet violet), *V.* spp., wild violet

WALNUT — *Juglans* spp.

WESTERN RED CEDAR — *Thuja plicata*

WHEAT — *Triticum x aestivum*

WILD GINGER — *Asarum canadense* (western variety)

WILD SARSAPARILLA — *Aralia nudicaulis*

WILD STRAWBERRY — *Fragaria virginiana, F. vesca*

WILLOW — *Salix* spp.

WISTERIA — *Wisteria* spp.

WITCH HAZEL — *Hammamelis virginiana*

WOLFBERRY — *Lycium chinense* (Chinese wolfberry)

WORMWOOD — *Artemisia absinthum* (absinthe)

YARROW — *Achilea millefolium* (woundwort, carpenter's herb)

YUCCA — *Yucca* spp.

One could say that the systematic naming of plants and animals is a form of biocentric chauvinism—that Man in all his vainglory has shepherded everything according to his needs into neat little categories—and this may be true to some degree. But I say that the careful observation of relationships between living beings, be they leafy, spiny, furry, feathery, leathery, or slithery, can be of great benefit to our understanding of each other as human beings and our connection to the wonderful world at large. Nature truly is the best teacher.

List of Recipes by Category

Home Remedies

Main Dishes

Nuts and Seeds

Salads and Relishes

Soups

Bibliography

Ackerman, Diane. *A Natural History of the Senses*. New York: Random House, 1990.

Aikman, Lonnelle. *Nature's Healing Arts*. Washington, D.C.: National Geographic Society, 1977.

American Society of Plant Biologists. "Early Origins of Maize in Mexico," 06/27/2008, www.biologynews.net.

Andrews, Tamra. *Nectar and Ambrosia — An Encyclopedia of Food in World Mythology*. Santa Barbara, CA: ABC-CLIO, Inc., 2000.

Andrews, Ted. *How to See and Read the Aura*. St. Paul, MN: Llewellyn Publications, 1991.

Bastianich, Lidia Matticchio. *Lidia's Italian-American Kitchen*. New York: Alfred A. Knopf, 2001.

Bianchini, Francesco, and Francesco Corbetta. *Fruits and Vegetables*. New York: Crown Publishers, Inc., 1975. (Originally published in 1973 by Arnoldo Mondadori.)

Biodisiac Institute. *The Biodisiac Book: Harnessing Nature's Organic Powers to Your Own Sexuality*. Mayfair, London: Arlington Books, Ltd., 1981.

Bricklin, Mark. *The Practical Encyclopedia of Natural Healing*. Emmaus, PA: Rodale Press, Inc., 1976.

Buchman, Dian Dincin. *The Complete Herbal Guide to Natural Health & Beauty*. Garden City, NY: Doubleday & Co., Inc., 1973.

— — —. *Dian Dincin Buchman's Herbal Medicine*. New York: Gramercy Publishing Company, 1979.

Campanelli, Pauline. *Wheel of the Year: Living the Magical Life*. St. Paul, MN: Llewellyn Publications, 1989.

Carini, Simona. "Variations on a Theme of Polenta," 2006, homepage.mac.com/scarini/Essay4.html.

Chessman, Andrea. *Summer in a Jar: Making Pickles, Jams & More.* Charlotte, VT: Williamson Publishing, 1985.

Chevallier, Andrew. *The Encyclopedia of Medicinal Plants.* London: Dorling Kindersley Ltd., 1996.

Chin, Wee Yeow, and Hsuan Keng. *An Illustrated Dictionary of Chinese Medicinal Herbs.* Sebastapol, CA: CRCS Publications, 1992.

Clark, Lewis J. *Lewis Clark's Field Guide to Wildflowers of Forest and Woodland in the Pacific Northwest.* Sydney, British Columbia: Gray's Publishing Ltd., 1974.

— — —. *Lewis Clark's Field Guide to Wildflowers of the Mountains in the Pacific Northwest.* Sydney, British Columbia: Gray's Publishing Ltd., 1975.

Clarkson, Rosetta E. *The Golden Age of Herbs and Herbalists.* New York: Dover Publications, 1972.

Clements, Frederic E., and Edith S. Clements. *Rocky Mountain Flowers.* New York: The H. W. Wilson Company, 1945.

Clute, Willard N. *The Common Names of Plants and Their Meanings.* Indianapolis, IN: Willard N. Clute & Co., 1942.

Cocconi, Emilio. *Liqueurs for All Seasons.* Wilton, CT: Lyceum Books, Inc., 1975. (Originally published in Milan by Fratelli Fabbri in 1974.)

Cook's Illustrated Magazine, ed. *The Best Kitchen Quick Tips.* Brookline, MA: America's Test Kitchen, 2003.

Coon, Nelson. *Using Plants for Healing.* Emmaus, PA: Rodale Press, 1963.

— — —. *Using Wild and Wayside Plants.* New York: Dover Publications, 1957.

Couch, Osma Palmer. *Basket Pioneering.* New York: Orange Judd Publishing Co., 1933.

Cowan, Eliot. *Plant Spirit Medicine.* Newberg, OR: Swan Raven & Company, 1995.

Craighead, John J., Frank C. Craighead, and Ray J. Davis. *A Field Guide to Rocky Mountain Wildflowers (from Northern Arizona and New Mexico to British Columbia).* Boston, MA: Houghton Mifflin Co., 1963.

Crocker, Pat. *The Healing Herbs Cookbook*. Toronto, Ontario: Robert Rose, Inc., 1999.

Crow, W. B. *The Occult Properties of Herbs and Plants*. New York: Samuel Weiser Inc., 1980.

Cruden, Loren. *Medicine Grove: A Shamanic Herbal*. Rochester, VT: Destiny Books, 1997.

Cullum, Elizabeth. *A Cottage Herbal*. North Pomfret, VT: David & Charles, Inc., 1975.

Culpepper, Nicholas. *Culpepper's Complete Herbal*. Slough, Berks, England: W. Foulsham & Co., Ltd., n.d.

Cunningham, Scott. *Cunningham's Encyclopedia of Magical Herbs*. St. Paul, MN: Llewellyn Publications, 1985.

— — —. *The Magic in Food: Legends, Lore & Spellwork*. St. Paul, MN: Llewellyn Publications, 1991.

— — —. *Magical Aromatherapy*. St. Paul, MN: Llewellyn Publications, 1989.

— — —. *Magical Herbalism*. St. Paul, MN: Llewellyn Publications, 1982.

Dampney, Janet, and Elizabeth Pomeroy. *All About Herbs*. New York: Simon & Schuster, Inc., 1985.

Davidow, Joie. *Infusions of Healing: Treasury of Mexican-American Herbal Remedies*. New York: Fireside, 1999.

Dawson, Ron. *Nature Bound Pocket Field Guide*. Boise, ID: OMNIgraphics Ltd., 1985.

Dayton, William A. *Notes on Western Range Forbs*. Washington, DC: Forest Service/USDA, 1960.

DeDominici, Eva. "Carmelite Water Recipe," 2008, www.recipezaar .com/recipe/print?id=252697.

Densmore, Frances. *How Indians Use Plants for Food, Medicine & Crafts*. New York: Dover Publications, Inc., 1974. (First published in 1928 by the U.S. Government Printing Office under the title *Uses of Plants by the Chippewa Indians*.)

Duff, Gail. *A Book of Pot-Pourri*. New York: Beaufort Books Publishers, 1985.

Duke, James A. *The Green Pharmacy*. Emmaus, PA: Rodale Press, 1977.

— — —. *Handbook of Edible Weeds*. Boca Raton, FL: CRC Press, 1992.

Durant, Mary. *Who Named the Daisy? Who Named the Rose?—A Roving Dictionary of North American Wildflowers*. New York: Dodd, Mead & Company, 1976.

Dweck, Anthony C. "Ethnobotanical Use of Plants, Part 4, The American Continent," www.dweckdata.com/Published_papers/American_ Indians.pdf.

Elliot, Doug. *Wild Roots*. Rochester, VT: Healing Arts Press, 1995.

Elpel, Thomas J. *Botany in a Day—Thomas J. Elpel's Herbal Field Guide to Plant Families*. Pony, MT: HOPS, 1996.

Frazer, Sir James G. *The Golden Bough*. New York: Touchstone, 1950.

Freitus, Joe. *Wild Preserves*. Boston, MA: Stonewall Press, Inc., 1977.

Gaines, Xerpha M., and D. G. Swan. *Weeds of Eastern Washington and Adjacent Areas*. Davenport, WA: Camp-Na-Bor-Lee Association, Inc., 1972.

Garland, Sarah. *The Complete Book of Herbs and Spices*. New York: The Viking Press, 1979.

Gibbons, Euell. *Stalking the Healthful Herbs*. New York: David McKay Company, Inc., 1966.

— — —. *Stalking the Wild Asparagus*. New York: David McKay Company, Inc., 1962.

Gilbertie, Sal. *Herb Gardening at Its Best*. New York: Athenaum/SM, 1978.

Gordon, Leslie. *Green Magic*. New York: Viking Press, 1977.

Graff, Ingrid. "Mint." *Blair & Ketchum's Country Journal*, March 1981.

Greene, Janet, Ruth Hertzberg, and Beatrice Vaughan. *Putting Food By*. New York: Penguin Group, 1992.

Grieve, Mrs. M. *A Modern Herbal—Volume I & II*. New York: Dover Publications, Inc., 1982. (Originally published in 1931 by Harcourt, Brace & Company.)

Griggs, Barbara. *Green Pharmacy: A History of Herbal Medicine*. New York: The Viking Press, 1981.

Gunther, Erna. *Ethnobotany of Western Washington*. Seattle: University of Washington Press, 1945.

Hart, Jeff. *Montana: Native Plants and Early Peoples*. Helena, MT: Montana Historical Society, 1976.

Hawken, Paul. *The Magic of Findhorn*. New York: Bantam, 1975.

Hazan, Marcella. *Essentials of Classic Italian Cooking*. New York: Alfred A. Knopf, 1995.

Heinerman, John. *Science of Herbal Medicine*. Orem, UT: Woodland Books, Bi-World Publishers, 1984.

Hersey, Jean. *A Woman's Day Book of Wildflowers*. New York: Fawcett Publications, 1960, 1976.

Hesse, Hermann. *Beneath the Wheel*. New York: Bantam, 1906, 1976.

Hickey, Michael, and Clive King. *The Cambridge Illustrated Glossary of Botanical Terms*. Cambridge, UK: Cambridge University Press, 2000.

Hillers, Val. *You Can Prevent Food Poisoning — PNW 250*. Washington State University/University of Idaho/Oregon State University/USDA, revised 1993.

Hitchcock, Leo C., and Arthur Cronquist. *Flora of the Pacific Northwest*. Seattle: University of Seattle Press, 1973.

Hole, John W., Jr. *Human Anatomy and Physiology*. Dubuque, IA: Wm. C. Brown Co., 1978, 1981.

Hopman, Ellen Evert. *A Druid's Herbal*. Rochester, VT: Destiny Books, 1995.

Hopping, Jane Watson. *The Pioneer Lady's Country Kitchen: A Seasonal Treasury of Time-Honored American Recipes*. New York: Villard Books, 1988.

Hutchens, Alma R. *Indian Herbalogy of North America*. Ontario, Canada: Merco, 1973.

Hylton, William H., ed. *The Rodale Herb Book*. Emmaus, PA: The Rodale Press, Inc., 1974.

Inglis, Bessie D. *Wild Flower Studies*. Great Britain: The Studio Publications, Inc., 1951.

Kanner, Catherine. *The Book of the Bath*. New York: Ballantine Books, 1985.

Katzen, Mollie. *The Moosewood Cookbook*. Berkeley, CA: Ten Speed Press, 1977.

Kavasch, Barrie. *American Indian Healing Arts*. New York: Bantam Books, 1999.

— — —. *Native Harvests: Recipes and Botanicals of the American Indian*. New York: Random House, Vintage Books, 1977.

Keville, Kathy. *The Illustrated Herb Encyclopedia*. New York: Mallard Press, 1991.

Kinucan, Edith S., and Penny R. Brons. *Wild Wildflowers of the West*. Ketchum, ID: Kinucan & Brons, 1977.

Kneipp, Sebastian. *My Water-Cure*. Mokelumne Hill, CA: Health Research, 1956. (First published in 1886 and translated from the 62nd German edition, Jos. Koessel, Publisher, Bavaria.)

Konowachuk, J., and J. I. Speirs. "Antiviral Effect of Apple Beverages." *Applied and Environmental Microbiology, Bureau of Microbial Hazards*. Ottawa, Ontario: Health and Welfare, Canada, 1978.

Kowalchik, Claire, and William H. Hylton, eds. *Rodale's Illustrated Encyclopedia of Herbs*. Emmaus, PA: Rodale Press, 1987.

Krause, Steven A. *Wine from the Wilds*. Harrisburg, PA: Stackpole Books, 1982.

Krompegel, Karla. "Ethnobotany of Two Contrasting American Ecosystems: Amazonia and the Sonoran Desert" (www.colostate.edu/Depts/Entomology/courses/en570/papers_2000/Krompegel.html).

Krutch, Joseph Wood. *Herbal*. Boston, MA: David R. Godine, Publisher, 1976.

Kushi, Aveline. *Aveline Kushi's Complete Guide to Macrobiotic Cooking*. New York: Warner Books, 1985.

Kynes, Sandra. *Whispers from the Woods: The Lore and Magic of Trees*. Woodbury, MN: Llewellyn Publications, 2006.

Larrison, Earl L., Grace W. Patrick, William H. Baker, and James A. Yaich. *Washington Wildflowers*. Seattle, WA: The Seattle Audobon Society, 1974.

Law, Donald. *Herbal Teas for Health and Pleasure*. Rustington, Sussex, England: Health Science Press, 1968.

Lawrence, George H. M. *An Introduction to Plant Taxonomy*. New York: The Macmillan Company, 1955.

Leek, Sybil. *Sybil Leek's Book of Herbs*. New York: Cornerstone Library, Simon & Shuster, 1973.

Levy, Juliette de Bairacli. *Common Herbs for Natural Health.* New York: Schocken Books, 1966, 1974.

Lust, John. *The Herb Book.* New York: Benedict Lust Publications, Bantam Books, 1974.

MacRae, Norma M. *Canning & Preserving Without Sugar.* Chester, CT: The Globe Pequot Press, 1982.

Malgieri, Nick. *How to Bake: The Complete Guide to Perfect Cakes, Cookies, Pies, Tarts, Breads, Pizzas, Muffins, Sweet and Savory.* New York: HarperCollinsPublications, 1995.

Marks, Geoffrey, and William K. Beatty. *The Medical Garden: Seven Important Drugs that Grow in the Wild.* New York: Charles Scribner's Sons, 1971.

Martha Stewart Living, eds. *The Martha Stewart Living Cookbook.* New York: Oxmoor House, 2000.

Martin, Laura C. *The Folklore of Trees and Shrubs.* Chester, CT: The Globe Pequot Press, 1992.

Meyer, David C., compiler. *Herbal Recipes.* Glenwood, IL: Meyerbooks, 1978.

Millspaugh, Charles F. *American Medicinal Plants.* New York: Dover Publications, Inc., 1974, unabridged republication. (Originally published in 1892 by John Yorston & Co., Philadelphia.)

Moerman, Daniel E. *American Medical Ethnobotany: A Reference Dictionary.* New York & London: Garland Publishing Inc., 1977.

———. *Geraniums for the Iroquois: A Field Guide to American Indian Medicinal Plants.* Algonac, MI: Reference Publications, Inc., 1981.

Moore, Michael. *Medicinal Plants of the Mountain West.* Santa Fe: The Museum of New Mexico Press, 1979.

———. *Medicinal Plants of the Pacific West.* Santa Fe: Red Crane Books, 1993.

Mowrey, Daniel B. *Proven Herbal Blends.* Ogden, UT: Root of Life, Inc., 1984.

Munson, Shirley, and Jo Nelson. *Apple Lover's Cook Book.* Phoenix, AZ: Golden West Publishers, 1995.

Niehaus, Theodore F., and Charles L. Ripper. *A Field Guide to Pacific States' Wildflowers.* The Peterson Field Guide Series. Boston: Houghton Mifflin Co., 1976.

Niethammer, Carolyn. *American Indian Food and Lore*. New York: Collier Books, Macmillan Publishing Co., Inc., 1974.

Olver, Lynne, ed., "History Notes: About Corn & Maize," 2008, www.foodtimeline.org/foodfaq.html.

Ornstein, Robert, and David Sobel. *Healthy Pleasures*. Reading, MA: Addison-Wesley, 1989.

Orr, Robert T., and Margaret C. Orr. *Wildflowers of Western America*. New York: Galahad Books, 1981.

Oster, Maggie, and Sal Gilbertie. *The Herbal Palate Cookbook*. Pownal, VT: Storey Communications, Inc., 1996.

Ott, John N. *Health and Light: The Effects of Natural and Artificial Light on Men and Other Living Things*. New York: Pocket Books, 1973.

Parvati, Jeannine. *Hygieia: A Woman's Herbal*. Monroe, UT: A Freestone Collective Book, 1978.

Passmore, Nancy F. W., ed. *The 1987 Lunar Calendar*. Boston, MA: Luna Press, 1986.

Patterson, Patricia A., et al. *Field Guide to Forest Plants of Northern Idaho*. Ogden, UT: USDA Forest Service, 1985.

Peltier, Jerome. *Manners and Customs of the Coeur d'Alene Indians*. Spokane, WA: Peltier Publications, 1975.

Peterson, Maude Gridley. *How to Know Wild Fruits*. New York: Dover Publications, Inc., 1973. (Unabridged republication of 1905 edition published by the Macmillan Company, new Table of Changes in Nomenclature by E. S. Harrar.)

Pickston, Margaret. *The Language of Flowers*. Facsimile Edition. Published in England by Michel Joseph Ltd., 1968.

Pond, Barbara. *A Sampler of Wayside Herbs: Rediscovering Old Uses for Familiar Wild Plants*. Riverside, CT: The Chatham Press, Inc., 1974.

Preston, Jr., Richard J. *Rocky Mountain Trees*. New York: Dover Publications, Inc., 1968. (Revised and corrected edition.)

Prindle, Tara. "Native American History of Corn," 2008, NativeTech: Native American Technology and Art, www.nativetech.org/cornhusk/cornhusk.html.

Pringle, Laurence. *Wild Foods*. New York: Four Winds Press, 1978.

Reavis, Charles. *Home Sausage Making*. Pownal, VT: Garden Way Publishing, 1981.

Rickett, Harold William. *Botany for Gardeners*. New York: The Macmillan Company, 1957.

Rodale, Robert, ed. "The Exciting World of Herbs," November 1977 special issue. Emmaus, PA: Rodale Press, Inc.

Rohde, Eleanour Sinclair. *A Garden of Herbs*. New York: Dover Publications, 1969.

Rombauer, Irma S. *Joy of Cooking*. New York: Simon & Schuster, 1977. (Originally self-published in 1931.)

Rose, Jeanne. *Herbs & Things*. New York: Perigee/Grosset & Dunlap, 1972.

— — —. *Jeanne Rose's Herbal Guide to Inner Health*. New York: Grosset & Dunlap, 1979.

— — —. *Jeanne Rose's Kitchen Cosmetics*. Los Angeles: Panjandrum Books, 1978.

Schmid, Ronald F. *Native Nutrition: Eating According to Ancestral Wisdom*. Rochester, VT: Healing Arts Press, 1987.

Schofield, Janis J. *Discovering Wild Plants*. Anchorage, AK: Alaska Northwest Books, 1989.

Sesti, Giuseppe Maria, et al. *The Phenomenon Book of Calendars*. New York: Phenomenon Publications Ltd., Simon & Schuster, 1978.

Seward, Barbara. *The Symbolic Rose*. Dallas, TX: Spring Publications, Inc., 1989.

Shababy, Doreen. "Wild & Weedy—A Journal of Herbology," Vol. 1, No. 1 through Vol. 6, No. 21 (1989–1995). Clark Fork, ID: self-published.

Shaudys, Phyllis V. *Herbal Treasures*. Pownal, VT: Garden Way Publishing, 1990.

— — —. *The Pleasure of Herbs*. Pownal, VT: Garden Way Publishing, 1986.

Smith, Jeff. *The Frugal Gourmet*. New York: Morrow, 1984.

Sokolov, Raymond. *With the Grain*. New York: Alfred A. Knopf, Inc., 1995

Spellenberg, Richard. T*he Audubon Society Field Guide to North American Wildflowers*. New York: Alfred A. Knopf, Inc., 1979.

Spoerke, Jr., David G. *Herbal Medications*. Santa Barbara, CA: Woodbridge Press Publishing Co., 1980.

Starhawk. *The Spiral Dance: A Rebirth of the Ancient Religion of the Great Goddess*. New York: Harper & Row, Publishers, Inc., 1979.

Stewart, Hilary. *Wild Teas, Coffees & Cordials: 60 Drinks of the Pacific Northwest*. Seattle: University of Washington Press, 1981.

Stuart, Malcolm, ed. *The Encyclopedia of Herbs and Herbalism*. London: Orbis Publishing Ltd., 1979.

Sun Bear, and Wabun. *The Medicine Wheel: Earth Astrology*. Englewood Cliffs, NJ: Prentice-Hall, Inc., 1980.

Sunset Magazine, eds. *Western Garden Book*. Menlo Park, CA: Sunset Publishing Corporation, 1992.

Sweet, Muriel. *Common Edible and Useful Plants of the West*. Healdsburg, CA: Naturegraph Company, 1962.

Symonds, George W. D. *The Tree Identification Book: A New Method for the Practical Identification and Recognition of Trees*. New York: William Morrow & Company, Inc., 1958.

Telesco, Patricia. *The Kitchen Witch's Cookbook*. St. Paul, MN: Llewellyn Publications, 1994.

Thiselton-Dyer, T. F. *The Folk-Lore of Plants*. Detroit, MI: Singing Trees Press, 1968. (Originally published in 1889 by Chatto & Windus, Piccadilly, London.)

Tilford, Gregory L. *The EcoHerbalist's Fieldbook*. Conner, MT: Mtn. Weed Publishing, 1993.

Time-Life Books. *Dried Beans & Grains*. The Good Cook Series. Alexandria, VA: Time-Life Books, 1980.

Tisserand, Maggie. *Aromatherapy for Women*. New York: Thorssons Publishers Inc., 1985.

Tisserand, Robert B. *The Art of Aromatherapy*. Rochester, VT: Healing Arts Press, 1977.

Tolley, Emelie, and Chris Mead. *The Herbal Pantry*. New York: Clarkson N. Potter, Inc., 1992.

Tompkins, Peter, and Christopher Bird. *The Secret Life of Plants*. New York: Avon Books, 1973.

Underhill, J. E. *Northwestern Wild Berries*. Surrey, British Columbia: Hancock House Publishers Ltd., 1980.

Vogel, Virgil J. *American Indian Medicine*. Norman, OK: The University of Oklahoma Press, 1970.

Wallace, Jim, and Maureen Wallace. *Snackers*. Seattle: Madrona Publishers, 1977.

Weber, William A. *Rocky Mountain Flora*. Boulder: Colorado Associated University Press, 1976.

Weed, Susun S. *Healing Wise*. Woodstock, NY: Ash Tree Publishing, 1989.

Weiner, Michael A. *Earth Medicine Earth Food*. New York: Fawcette Columbine, 1972.

Weiss, Gaea, and Shandor Weiss. *Growing & Using the Healing Herbs*. Emmaus, PA: Rodale Press, 1985.

Welsh, Stanley L., and B. Ratcliffe. *Flowers of the Mountain Country*. Provo, UT: Brigham Young University Press, 1975.

Went, Frits W. *The Plants*. New York: Time, Inc., 1973.

White, Linda R., and Sunny Mavor. *Kids, Herbs & Health*. Loveland, CO: Interweave Press, 1998.

Will, George F., and George E. Hyde. *Corn Among the Indians of the Upper Missouri*. Lincoln and London: University of Nebraska Press, 1964.

Williamson, Darcy. *How to Prepare Common Wild Foods*. 1978, self-published.

Witkowski, Desirée. *The Passionate Palate: Recipes for Cooking up a Delicious Life*. St. Paul, MN: Llewellyn Publications, 1999.

Witty, Helen. *Fancy Pantry*. New York: Workman Publishing, 1986.

Wolfert, Paula. *The Cooking of the Eastern Mediterranean: 215 Healthy, Vibrant and Inspired Recipes*. New York: HarperCollinsPublishers, 1994.

— — —. *The Cooking of South-West France: A Collection of Traditional and New Recipes from France's Magnificent Rustic Cuisine, and New Techniques to Lighten Hearty Dishes*. Garden City, NY: The Dial Press, Doubleday & Company, Inc., 1983.

Yemm, J. R., ed. *The Medical Herbalist*. No. Hollywood, CA: Wilshire Book Company, 1976.

Yocom, Charles, Vinson Brown, and Aldine Starbuck. *Wildlife of the Intermountain West*. Healdsburg, CA: Naturegraph Publishers Inc., 1958

zana. "Precious Oils: Making Sun-Infused Healing Oils from Herbs." *WomanSpirit Magazine*, Summer Solstice, Vol. 10, No. 40, 1984. Wolf Creek, OR.

Index